Technological Innovations for Effective Pandemic Response

This reference text discusses the potential of efficient R&D management during times of pandemic crisis and how it can provide time-bound real-life deliverables to ward off the contamination-linked vulnerability aspects of social interaction.

It discusses important topics including mechanical ventilators with oxygen enrichment, hospital waste management facilities, hospital care assistive robotic devices, implementation of smart manufacturing, special purpose machines, micromachining, 3D printing, disposal of plastic waste utilizing high temperature plasma, automatic biomass briquetting plants and fully automatic biodiesel plants.

Features:

- Discusses novel technological innovations developed especially to effectively counter pandemics such as COVID-19.
- Explores how R&D modeling of technology can be interspersed with socioeconomic values.
- Covers how innovative technological solutions can be developed as per the situational requisites and deployed in the least possible time to make maximum impact.
- Discusses industrial manufacturing and automation techniques.

The text will be useful for graduate students and academic researchers working in diverse areas such as mechanical engineering, industrial engineering, production engineering, manufacturing science and automobile engineering.

It covers influences of pandemics on water and sanitation services, floating capsule-based biofilm reactor (FCBBR) methodology and innovative segregation of waste through a mechanized model.

Technological Innovations for Effective Pandemic Response

Harish Hirani

CRC Press
Taylor & Francis Group
Boca Raton London New York

CRC Press is an imprint of the
Taylor & Francis Group, an **informa** business

CRC Press
Boca Raton and London

First edition published 2022
by CRC Press
6000 Broken Sound Parkway NW, Suite 300, Boca Raton, FL 33487-2742

and by CRC Press
4 Park Square, Milton Park, Abingdon, Oxon, OX14 4RN
CRC Press is an imprint of Taylor & Francis Group, LLC

ISBN: 9781032312187 (hbk)
ISBN: 9781032362939 (pbk)
ISBN: 9781003331179 (ebk)

DOI: 10.1201/9781003331179

Typeset in Sabon
by Deanta Global Publishing Services, Chennai, India

Contents

Figures

Author's note

COVID-19 has put a number of restrictions on our economic and social life; and this pandemic has been a test of resilience for humanity at large. Scientifically improved resource utilization, fast learning from experiences and tackling big problems through a series of small solutions have been some of the major learnings from COVID-19. The book *Technological Innovations for Effective Pandemic Response* aptly recreates how the human mind, when deployed rationally, can deliver results unprecedented in recent history.

Public funded R&D institutes, being science and technology organizations, are supposed to incessantly study and understand the lacunas of the existent technologies and deliver effective solutions to the evolving needs of society. Thus, rearranging work and talent to build resilience to ensure time-bound translation of anti-pandemic R&D became the first priority for research institutions. This essentially meant priority-linked delivery of cost-effective technologies for immediate deployment. As the nature of the guidelines and protocols keep on changing, the developed technologies get modified and value-added in the form of different versions. The book describes how a public-funded organization can outperform by channelizing its resources effectively.

The most challenging part of developing a technology and deploying it for usage of the society during the lockdown phase is the lack of proper supply chain logistics. This aberration can be managed by promoting a local level approach, skilling/reskilling/upskilling workers to fit in their jobs, creating a more nimble and innovative economy through innovative usage of available resources in a cost-effective manner throughout the ecosystem. Encouraging everyone to enhance their skills ultimately makes the nation more competitive in the global market.

The public–private partnership and pricing profile of the technologies ensure maximum participation of the micro and small entrepreneurs, and through their participation, the outreach of the technology to the society is also ensured. Besides, the innovative yet simple design formulation of the technologies to suit available resources and partnering with different organizations enable the raw materials for the technology to be easily sourced and manufactured at any location. This provides an opportunity to transform society in ways that reduce inequality and generate gainful employment for thousands of the young workforce across the nation. This pandemic taught us importance of "localized water collection, sanitation and purification", "localized safe disposal of municipal waste", "robotics and digitization in healthcare units", "low-cost automation of agricultural machinery", and "strong local level administration" as part of the "social protection strategy". It is also ensured that the anti-pandemic technologies are clean, green and carbon neutral and thus emphasis is to be given to harness renewable sources of energy. The three major constituents of the environment, i.e., air, water and solid waste are to be appropriately addressed through the developed technologies to ensure that a pristine and hygienic environment is maintained throughout. The available financial resources are to be deployed in a manner to ensure maximum result through the carefully curated concept of "impact investment".

The author personally was taken aback to a certain extent just a few days before the onset of the COVID-19 pandemic in India by a severe lung infection. Even though maximum rest was suggested by the doctors for full recovery, the COVID-19 pandemic demanded immediate attention. We, being practitioners of science and technology, have a certain degree of responsibility toward the society, especially so during a crisis such as this, which is beyond any selfish ideation. Thus, it was my solemn duty to ensure that the R&D institution headed by me stood up to its principal motto, i.e., "Maximum Science for Minimum Societal and Ecological Distress".

Preface

Pandemics have been wreaking havoc on human civilization since ages and have always been at crossroads with the progress of human civilization. SARS-CoV-2 and Spanish flu are just testimonies to what awaits us in the future. Such pandemics bring public health issues, medical challenges, large scale economic crises and social instability. As was the case in Wuhan, China, in November 2019, viruses inevitably mutate themselves into multiple form factors and become extremely lethal for the human race. The COVID-19 pandemic has ravaged the foundations of the global economy and has destroyed the fundamentals of human social interaction (*no-gathering in-person, no handshakes, no hugs*), owing to its extremely transmittable nature. There is a need to use scientific and technical methodologies to control the virus and minimize its spreading capabilities, alleviate human suffering and catalyze economic recovery.

Every pandemic is different, yet there are a number of common doses of humility and humanity (i.e., *collective decision-making, curiosity and open-mindedness, voluntarily limiting activity to avoid getting sick, deploying all available tools to avoid economic recession*) to deal with the health and economic shocks. The maximum collateral damage inflicted usually occurs during the stage of developing the initial form of the vaccine and thus a protective shield (*wearing mask, sanitizing surroundings, avoiding meeting in-person*) needs to be adopted to ensure that the vulnerable sections of the community are protected from the associated devastation. This is where engineering can step in and play the role of a powerful sentinel to arrest the transmission of the disease through carefully curated affordable technologies. The supply chain may also be attuned in a manner, to ensure seamless flow of necessary inputs and a robust logistics gateway for smooth delivery of services, during the stressed-out period of pandemics. Thus, engineering and medical science can work hand-in-hand to achieve the stated goals instead of being at loggerheads with each other. A strategic approach involving the localized solid, liquid and hospital waste management and a complete protection system for gated societies and hospitals at local levels to suppress the spread of virus to the lowest possible level to return to normal life ASAP has been detailed.

A collaborative economic framework has also been carefully crafted in the later chapters of this book, which illustrates how the economy of a particular society can be designed and positioned so that it is able to counter all the sluggishness and slowdowns which are usually associated with a pandemic-like situation. This can be achieved by a significant shift in behavior: "individualism to interdependence", "competitiveness to collaboration" and "eliminating deceiving nature". The individuals can be motivated to follow social norms by minimizing "pandemic fear" by publicizing scientific findings on "effective solutions to combat pandemic" and that is the aim of this book. New kinds of industries on waste management, recycling of waste resources, solar energy, air purification, irrigation and soil and water conservation with appropriate business models for unemployed people and micro–small enterprises have been suggested. It is essential for all to come together and join hands to defeat the pandemic and for that purpose the science by local authorities for society (SLS) model, where the collaboration of the state and the residents results in a better provision of sanitation services and accountability, is proposed considering the increase in the "happiness quotient" by conducting collaborative social activities. The economic framework tries to emulate a cyclical and sustainable economy model which can endure/withstand the crisis-related stresses. This will help in maintaining the economic momentum, which consequently will help sustain the economy.

It is known that food is an essential item for everyone; the integrated agriculture (farming, farm machinery, manufacturing, water management, waste management) sector has to see a growth in the post pandemic scenario minimizing the unemployment rates in the sector. Furthermore, as the young generation loves automation, the automated and digital farming would attract them to this field.

Acknowledgments

This book is a testimony to how time-bound and sociocentric translation of R&D can make a massive difference in times of unprecedented crisis such as the pandemic. The technologies listed in the book can make tremendous socioeconomic impact across the nation and can provide hundreds of families a sustainable alternative for income generation during a time of such unprecedented economic crisis.

I take this opportunity to express my gratitude to Dr. Amit Ganguly and Mr. Partha Das for efforts toward development of the solid and liquid waste management and mechanized drain cleaning technology, Dr. Poulomi Roy and Dr. Himadri Roy for design and development of all variants of face-masks, Dr. Bittagopal Mandal for his efforts toward the development of the 360° car flusher, Shri S.R. Debbarma and Dr. Chanchal Loha for their efforts toward the development of disinfection walkways, Dr. R.P. Barnwal for his efforts toward development of the IntelliMAST, Shri Avinash Yadav for his efforts toward development of the BPDS, Dr. Malay Karmakar for his efforts toward development of the POMID, Dr. Anupam Sinha for his efforts toward development of the mechanical ventilators, Dr. Priyabrata Banerjee for his efforts toward development of the hospital waste management system, Shri Subho Samanta for his efforts toward development of the dry fogging shoe disinfector, Dr. Anjali Chatterjee and Dr. A. Maity for their efforts toward development of the HCARD, Dr. S.R.K. Vadali for his efforts toward development of the touchless faucet, Dr. L.G. Das and Dr. Palash Maji for their efforts toward development of the road sanitizer unit, Dr. Sarita Ghosh for her efforts toward development of the basic liquid soap, Dr. Tapas Kuila for his efforts toward development of the hand sanitizers and Dr. Vadali and Shri J.P. Maji for their efforts toward development of the soap dispenser. Author acknowledges the contributions of Dr. Sudip Kumar Samanta, Dr. Manidipto Mukherjee, Mr. S.Y. Pujar, Mr. Ved Prakash, Mr. Balaji Chandrakanth, Mr. Sourav Halder, Dr. Arup Nandi and Mr. Avinash Yadav of Council of Scientific and Industrial Research-Central Mechanical Engineering Research Institute (CSIR-CMERI), Durgapur, including Dr. Barnali Mondal of NIT Durgapur in writing the chapter on manufacturing.

I would also like to thank Dr. Sarita Ghosh, Shri Amrit Kumar, Shri Rajshekar Ghosh and Dr. Biplab Choudhury for assisting in the compilation of this book. I express my special and sincere gratitude to all the members of the CSIR-CMERI family, whose collective efforts made the technological breakthroughs possible.

Harish Hirani

Author

Dr. Harish Hirani is presently a professor in IIT Delhi. He has more than 140 research publications and 140 IPR (granted/applied) to his credit. His book on "Fundamentals of Engineering Tribology with Applications", published by Cambridge University Press has proven to be a success. He is Fellow of the Institute of Engineers (FIE) and a member of ASME. He has organized and conducted more than 25 training courses for 1000+ engineering faculties and 300+ industry executives. With a robust research experience of more than 25 years, 20+ years of teaching experience in IITs, more than eight years of academic and scientific administrative experience and six months of research experience at Massachusetts Institute of Technology, Cambridge, USA, Prof Hirani always strived to inculcate the culture of spreading scientific awareness/technological innovations among scientists/researchers and learners for realizing substantial socioeconomic impact.

He was Director of CSIR-Central Mechanical Engineering Research Institute (CMERI) from 16.03.2016 to 15.03.2022. He is a firm believer of inclusive growth and paves the ways of technology transfer to micro and small enterprises so that common people are benefited. Even in the crucial time of COVID-19, a number of technologies/products were developed to benefit the society. In his opinion, the technologies invented at government intuitions can be translated into economic, user-friendly, high-quality solutions; therefore, a paradigm shift in attitude and action of scientists is the need of the hour to match with the dynamic highly competitive industry thriving on innovative solutions. There is a need to spread scientific awareness and use science of management economics to help farmers and small-scale manufacturing industries and appropriately guide and motivate young minds to build a prosperous and self-reliant society.

Chapter 1

Current scenario of the pandemic and challenges

On 31.12.2019, the World Health Organization (WHO) was informed about a new type of pneumonia disease diagnosed in Wuhan City, China. On 07.01.2020, China identified coronavirus as the cause of the disease. The WHO named this virus as SARS-CoV-2 and the disease as COVID-19. As per WHO [1], more than 1.27 million people died in less than one year of COVID-19 disease. The novel coronavirus SARS-CoV-2 is the seventh member of the Coronaviridae family of viruses which are enveloped, non-segmented, positive-sense RNA viruses [2]. Fortunately, the mortality rate of COVID-19 is less than that of the severe acute respiratory syndrome (SARS) and Middle East respiratory syndrome (MERS) coronavirus diseases, but SARS-CoV-2 is highly infectious [3]. The transmission of SARS-CoV-2 can occur via respiratory secretions [4]. It is considered that the viral respiratory infection not only spreads by direct contact, but may also spread through droplet transmission. The droplets released during coughing and sneezing may be of different sizes, larger ones with 0.1 mm or more and the smaller droplets with size <10 μm [5]. Researchers found that viruses may remain infectious in aerosols for 3 hours or more [6].

This pandemic has significantly disrupted the global economic scenario and increased unemployment throughout. The economic stress is impacting the relationship difficulties and changing the content of social interactions and affecting the psychological state of the society at large. In such cases, the assistance provided by government may not be enough; there is an urgent need to address social and economic problems and provide a SMART (Specific, Measurable, Achievable, Realistic, Time Bound) solution.

Human civilization has been disrupted by pandemics (i.e., plague, cholera, SARS, MERS, flu, etc.) quite regularly through its history, though the scale of devastation has been different. Some of the most ravaging pandemics in human history are: the "Great Plague of London 1665", "Russian Flu 1889", "Spanish Flu 1918" and "Asian Flu 1957". Thus, owing to the recurrence of pandemics of such scale, it is very important for the human society at large to be prepared to combat the ravaging effects of such health emergencies through resilient economic frameworks powered by technology-driven innovations and human willpower. This book proposes

DOI: 10.1201/9781003331179-1

a holistic framework of tackling the impact of future pandemics through a carefully devised multi-pronged strategy.

1.1 SCIENCE, TECHNOLOGY AND INNOVATION FOR TACKLING PANDEMIC

Insight into science and technology related to pandemic in terms of "aligning human behavior", "public health", and "techno-economics" together will be very much useful to tackle the pandemic. Council of Scientific and Industrial Research (CSIR) is known for dissemination and application of science and technology. CSIR has 37 national laboratories which can be categorized into two broad categories: pharma and non-pharma laboratories. Pharma laboratories mostly focus on development of medicine, vaccines and testing technologies. Testing of antibodies related to pandemic disease is essential to differentiate between active and non-active cases. For example, reverse transcription-polymerase chain reaction (RT-PCR) is being used to test COVID-19. In this method of testing, a nasal/throat swab is used to extract ribonucleic acid or RNA (the genetic material of the virus) from a patient. If it shares the same genetic sequence as SARS-CoV-2 virus, then it is deemed positive [7]. The negative test means the actual sample, extracted from the concerned person, does not carry the virus, but there is also a possibility that the test was not administered properly. An alternative approach, in case of COVID-19, is the use of computed tomography (CT) imaging, which is a non-invasive test conducted to obtain a precise image of a patient's chest [8], giving physicians a better view for making accurate diagnoses.

Non-pharma laboratories develop various solutions targeting the reduction of spread of the virus. To quantify the spread of pandemic disease, reproduction number R0 (the average number of additional people infected by each infected person) is used. The growing value of R0 can be reduced by imposing lockdown, testing and quarantine measures so that spreading from infected persons can be minimized. The R0 should be less than 0.8 to ensure the epidemic reduces and ultimately dies out. The use of masks/protective equipment and measurement of body temperature using infrared thermography are well known to limit the virus spread. As it is known that the virus is transmitted from person to person through respiratory droplets or contact, it is advisable to increase hand washing and use of facemasks in public, and in this regard, researchers of non-pharma laboratories are supposed to find alternative resources to minimize the effect of "panic buying" and "stocking up on supplies" behavior of the people so that marginalized communities get the required supply. There is a need for a shift in behavior: "individualism to interdependence", "competitiveness to collaboration" and "eliminating deceiving nature". The individuals can be motivated to obey social norms through minimizing "pandemic fear" by publicizing scientific findings on "effective solutions to combat pandemic" and that is the aim of this book. New kinds of industries on waste management, recycling of waste resources, solar energy, air purification, irrigation and soil and water conservation with appropriate business models for unemployed people and micro–small enterprises have been suggested to attain a degree of economic sustainability during such times.

1.2 LOCAL-LEVEL MANAGEMENT FOR WATER, SANITATION, HYGIENE AND WASTE

As per WHO, the facility of water, sanitation, hygiene and safe disposal of wastes are essential for preventing and protecting human health during all infectious disease outbreaks [9], including COVID-19. As per the estimates provided by WHO and UNICEF, around three billion people lack hand sanitation facilities at home globally. Lack of sanitation causes several million deaths around the world and therefore it is very important to ensure appropriate hand washing and waste disposal culture in communities, homes, schools, marketplaces and hospitals to prevent transmission of pathogens including SARS-CoV-2, and consequently, there is a need to involve local initiatives to combat pandemic. Local-level manufacturing and innovations to meet the enormous demand of products like liquid soaps, masks, and sanitizers and that too in a cost-effective manner are essential. The manufactured products need to fulfill the primary requirements of functional performance and complementary performance requirements (i.e., useful life, reliability, simple to use, easy maintenance, etc.).

Innovations in developing "touchless faucet to cater to the frequent need of washing hands with soap and water", "energy efficient soap dispenser", "precision disinfection walkway", "cost-effective disinfection walkway", "road sanitizing unit", "battery powered disinfectant sprayer", "360° car flusher", "dry fogging shoe disinfector", etc. are found to be the need of the hour. All these technologies will surely reduce R0 in any locality of the world. The developed technologies can be customized/upgraded as per the requirement. As per the advisories from WHO, the spraying of sodium hypochlorite on people walking through a disinfectant tunnel may be harmful. In other words, there are some chances of having harmful effects if the solution of sodium hypochlorite is sprayed on the body [10]. Local-level programs to handle various pandemic situations, due to their flexibility, must be encouraged as these measures become more effective than the centralized methods. Proponents to local-level management can be successful in pursuing sustainability to combat pandemic.

Cleaning of drainage/sewage systems through manual scavenging is a conventional practice which violates the principles of human dignity and hygiene standards. The manual scavenging often creates small cracks in the sewage piped network, which can lead to contaminating the intermittent piped water supplied to various communities. Study also suggests that the deadly coronavirus can thrive in untreated water [11]. This book describes a mechanized drainage cleaning system and on-site waste water purification technologies to show the possibility of waste water treatment as an inseparable aspect of the water purification architecture in the near future. The decentralized approaches for wastewater reuse and improvements in local environmental health conditions have been recommended. Mobile drainage cleaning systems to suck water and purify it by passing through sieve membrane filtration by deploying technological innovation has been explained.

1.3 RECOVERY PATH

What is the likely recovery path of growth under a pandemic situation? The best method is to face the pandemic head-on and try to contain and mitigate the disease itself by introducing/utilizing various technologies. It is worth mentioning that each pandemic is unpredictable, so instead of going to the survival mode, one needs to opt for a learning mode. Learning is the foundation of survival. One needs to employ an iterative but scientific approach to understand, respond and learn lessons from rapidly unfolding events. Therefore, a high degree of innovation, deployment of technologies for a range of products and services provided may be the right methodology for socioeconomic recovery from a pandemic hit situation.

IMF projections suggest that the economic recession caused by COVID-19 will be "far worse" than the Great Recession of 2008–2009 [12]. This recession seems to be severe for the smaller businesses and farmers. To deal with financial crisis and recession, there is a need to work on small business and innovate user-friendly agricultural affordable machinery. It is known that food is an essential item for everyone; the agriculture sector has to see a growth in the post pandemic scenario minimizing the unemployment rates in the sector. Furthermore, as the young generation loves automation, automated and digital farming would attract them to this field. To support micro, small and medium enterprises (MSMEs) and marginalized farmers, a number of agricultural machineries such as smaller 9 to 12 HP tractors, pneumatic precision planters for vegetables, inter-row rotary cultivators for wide-row crops, offset rotavators for orchards, programmable irrigation schedulers, solar energy-based automatic irrigation systems, tractor front-mounted Mentha harvesters, controlled atmosphere renewable (biomass/solar) energy-based stand-alone cold storage ginger/turmeric processing technology: washing, slicing, drying, automatic biomass briquetting plants, oil expeller technologies (1–10 TPD), fully automatic biodiesel plants, leaf collector and shredding machines, conversion of horticulture waste into briquettes, biogas from grass/weeds, etc. can be developed. In addition to farm machinery, allied areas like the proposed First Generation E-Tractors, generation of surplus solar energy, need of farm mechanization for major crops, excellence in design and manufacturing of solar cooking systems, mechanism to check the wastage in perishable fruits and vegetables, etc. may prove to be a game changer toward enhancing the income of the farmers and microindustries.

1.4 OUTLINE

Pandemics have always been at crossroads with the progress of human civilization. During the initial stage of developing the vaccine, a veritable front needs to be formed against the invisible enemy to help citizens maintain high levels of hygiene to ensure that the vulnerable sections of the community are protected from the associated devastation. This is where engineering can step in and play the role of a powerful sentinel, whose role would be to contain the transmission of the disease through carefully curated affordable technologies, medical devices, pandemic awareness and best practices for a safe work environment. The engineering solutions, such as value-added facemasks, tractor-mounted road sanitization units, disinfection walkways, hospital waste management systems, touchless soap-cum-water dispensing units, hospital care assistive robotic devices (HCARDs), etc. must be launched for welfare of the society and to slow down the effect of the invisible enemy of the mankind. Special emphasis must be given to supply chains in terms of changing labor and material availabilities, shifting markets and transportation hindrance. The "use and throw" model where consumers discard products permanently must be discouraged. The supply chain may also be attuned in a manner to ensure seamless flow of necessary inputs and a robust logistics gateway for smooth delivery of services, during the stressed-out period of pandemics.

Chapter 3 of this book emphasizes on effective strategies for immediate deployment of appropriate civic management at the local level to fortify resilience toward countering the pandemic menace. The new model for strategy development related to municipal solid and liquid wastes, resource allocation and managing performance to handle the pandemic scenario and creating a pandemic resilient ecology is explained.

Every pandemic situation brings not only a period of global health issues but also a time-span of significant economic crisis. Such a recession rapidly increases unemployment in many countries. Many companies suffer enormously due to ongoing expenses and little or no revenue and face the grim prospect of never reopening. Many unemployed youths would like to start their own micro or small business depending on their financial strength. Chapter 4 of this book describes the role of individuals, public R&D organizations, non-governmental organizations (NGOs) and government agencies to act together with a sense of urgency and with prudence. An economic framework can be carefully crafted to illustrate how the economy of a particular society can be positioned so that it is able to counter all the sluggishness and slowdowns which are usually associated with a pandemic situation.

Engineering and manufacturing can go hand in hand to develop new products and create an ecosystem, which is aptly capable of responding to any future pandemic scenario through a multi-pronged approach. New opportunities for manufacturing sectors must be focused on. This has been explained in Chapter 5 of the book. It will help in maintaining an economic momentum, which consequently will help sustain the economy.

BIBLIOGRAPHY

1. https://covid19.who.int/, 2020
2. David S. Hui, Esam I. Azhar, Tariq A. Madani, Francine Ntoumi, Richard Kock, Osman Dar, Giuseppe Ippolito, Timothy D. Mchugh, Ziad A. Memish, Christian Drosten, et al. The continuing 2019-nCoV epidemic threat of novel coronaviruses to global health—the latest 2019 novel coronavirus outbreak in Wuhan, China. *International Journal of Infectious Diseases*, 91:264, 2020.
3. Heshui Shi, Xiaoyu Han, Nanchuan Jiang, Yukun Cao, Osamah Alwalid, Jin Gu, Yanqing Fan, and Chuansheng Zheng. Radiological findings from 81 patients with COVID-19 pneumonia in Wuhan, China: a descriptive study. *The Lancet Infectious Diseases*, 20(4): 425–434, 2020.
4. https://www.nhp.gov.in/coronavirus-infection_pg, 2020
5. Leung, N.H.L., Chu, D.K.W., Shiu, E.Y.C. *et al.* Respiratory virus shedding in exhaled breath and efficacy of face masks. *Nature Medicine*, 26: 676–680, 2020, DOI: 10.1056/NEJMc2004973
6. van Doremalen, N., Bushmaker, T., Morris, Dylan H., Holbrook, Myndi G ., Gamble, A. et al. Aerosol and Surface Stability of SARS-CoV-2 as Compared with SARS-CoV-1. *The New England Journal of Medicine*, 382(16): 1564–1567, 2020, DOI: 10.1056/NEJMc2004973.
7. https://www.thehindu.com/sci-tech/science/covid-19-what-are-the-different-types-of-tests/article31507970.ece, 2020
8. https://www.ncbi.nlm.nih.gov/pmc/articles/PMC8545281, 2020
9. https://www.who.int/publications/i/item/WHO-2019-nCoV-IPC-WASH-2020.4, 2020
10. https://www.aninews.in/news/national/general-news/use-of-sodium-hypochlorite-may-have-harmful-effects-aiims-d-doctor20200501202033/#:~:text=Use%20of%20sodium%20hypochlorite%20may%20have%20harmful%20effects%3A%20AIIMS%2DD%20Doctor,-ANI%20%7C%20Updated%3A%20May&text=Now%20sodium%20hypochlorite%20is%20a,%2C%22%20Dr%20Singh%20told%20ANI, 2020
11. Poulomi Roy. *Waste Water Treatment: An Unavoidable Solution to COVID-19*. CSIR-CMERI, Durgapur, 2021.
12. https://en.wikipedia.org/wiki/COVID-19_recession, 2020

Chapter 2

Innovative technological interventions to combat pandemic proliferation

Human civilization has been disrupted by pandemics quite regularly through its history, though the scale of devastation has been different. There is a strong relation between pandemic and virus. "Containment of virus", "disinfecting virus" and "medical help to recover from viral disease" are the "effective solutions to combat a pandemic". Expectation of complete help to be provided by government may not be correct and there is a need to address social and economic problems by society itself. This can be achieved by promoting "individualism to interdependence" and "competitiveness to collaboration" in every individual. Further intervention from scientists on "development of vaccine and rapid testing facilities/kits, formulation of drugs, manufacturing of devices to reduce spread of the virus, disinfection for the virus, healthcare, etc." and strict precautionary measures from every part of the society are expected.

Every pandemic is different. Even after the best efforts, the development of a comprehensive vaccine may require 6–18 months' clinical trials to prove its efficacy. Therefore, efforts toward the development of an array of small protective/precautionary intervention technologies such as healthcare assistive devices, value-added facemasks, tractor-mounted road sanitization units, disinfection walkways, hospital waste management systems, touchless soap-cum-water dispensing units, hospital care assistive robotic devices (HCARDs), etc. should be made, which, when synchronized collectively, can work as a veritable front against the spread of the lethal virus. In pandemic situations, the S&T community works tirelessly to bring in technological solutions, such as above, for tackling the danger of the pandemic and helping the society. From an engineering point of view, various actions as shown in Figure 2.1 can be conceptualized.

Figure 2.1 may be useful for individuals and organizations (i.e., schools, marketplaces, hospitals) to design objects, services and environments having technological solutions and prevent people from transmission of pathogens including SARS-CoV-2. Developing products/services by users has always been rewarding for society, as production and consumption need not be separated, and there are opportunities for improvements, customizations, complements and becoming self-sustainable. Such a "do

DOI: 10.1201/9781003331179-2

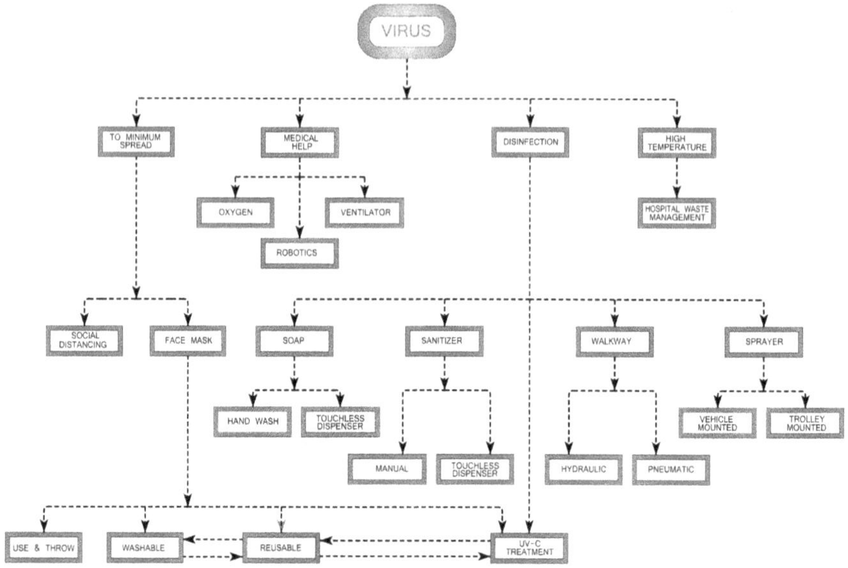

Figure 2.1 Pandemic resilience through protective technologies.

it yourself (DIY)" approach can create a stable economy and can generate employment for the jobless while serving society. Such an approach is required to create a positive social environment and pave the way for sustainable community.

One important point to be noticed from Figure 2.1 is that users can define the need and proceed with solution(s) based on the available local resources. However, during a pandemic, a major challenge is "time constraint"; therefore, in the rest of the chapter, knowledge and concepts of the required products to control the pandemic/epidemic have been described. With the use of these concepts, individuals/organizations can develop products in a short span of time and can create programs to train senior residents and unemployed youngsters for their economic sustenance.

2.1 FACEMASK

Wearing of facemasks as a piece of personal protective equipment (PPE) is highly desirable not only for the frontline workers but also for the common people. If worn properly, masks may be effective in preventing transmission of any epidemic such as flu, influenza, coronavirus, etc. During a pandemic, the need for facemasks increases significantly, which causes a global shortage of the item. Fortunately, facemasks are the easiest to fabricate.

2.1.1 Best practice approaches to implement specific behavioral interventions

Different kinds of facemasks ranging from both high-end N95 respirator masks to lower-end cotton/other fabric masks are in use. An N95 facemask with better fitting is highly recommended to stop very small particles. However, efficient filtration of airborne particles by the N95 facemask depends on the very close facial fit, which is often difficult to manufacture in local regions. Therefore, surgical masks or similar types of masks, which are easy to manufacture, dominate the market. There is a need to follow the general guidelines, as depicted in Figure 2.2, while wearing a facemask to reduce the chances of inhaling water particles containing the virus. The general guidelines of wearing facemasks comprise (a) disinfecting hands using a soap solution/sanitizer, (b) holding the facemask with their strings (and strictly not by their surface), (c) holding the facemask by the strings using both the hands, (d) ensuring complete covering of the face, i.e., mouth and nose to be covered. The most inappropriate method of wearing a facemask is either letting the facemask hang loosely below the nose while walking or letting it hang down the chin while talking. Such incorrect methods sometimes lead to a rapid spread of the epidemic.

2.1.2 Facemasks – the reusability factor

A recent report [1] says that wearing of surgical masks reduces the overall viral RNA copies in exhaled breath and cough aerosols by 3.4-folds. With a rapid increase in the public usage of facemasks, the demand for mask

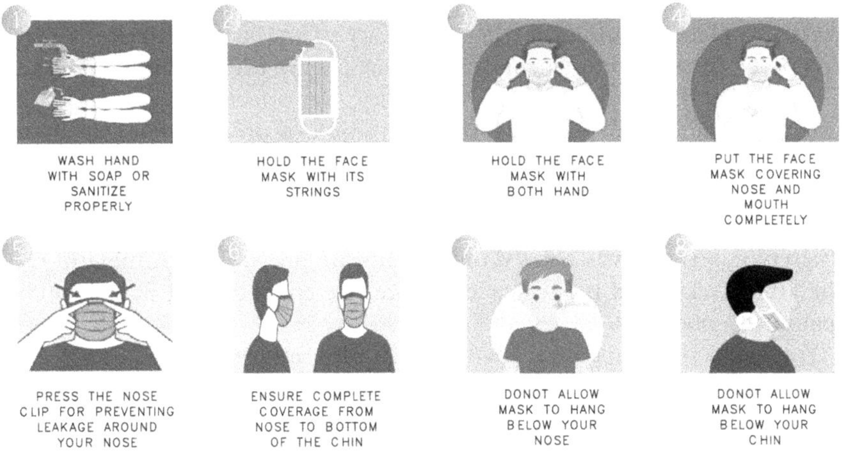

Figure 2.2 General guidelines for wearing facemasks.

reusability emerges, as the potential risk of unsafe disposal of facemasks can increase the chances of contamination and transmission. To minimize the waste created by surgical masks, reusable masks from hydrophobic non-woven polypropylene (PP) fabric can be fabricated. The approach of (a) using reusable facemasks and (b) sanitizing the mask after every single use may reduce the potential danger caused by unsafe disposal of facemasks. The term "reusable" refers to washing the facemasks regularly without damaging the efficiency of protection. UV-C rays can also be utilized to sanitize the facemasks that are difficult to wash.

The scientifically designed cost-effective facemask [2, 3] requires a total techno-economic solution. Three-layered protection-efficient facemasks can be developed using washable non-woven polypropylene (PP) fabric to restrict the contaminated droplets from entering or from being transmitted from one person to another. To enhance the filtration efficiency (to restrict sub-micrometer particulates effectively), the middle layer of the mask is to be made of a "high efficiency particulate air" filter. This kind of reusable and cost-effective mask is an effective barrier and prevents transmission of bacteria/viruses inward/outward.

One of the most important features of a facemask is the hydrophobicity (water-repelling nature of mask material). The test procedure to find hydrophobicity (water-repelling ability/wettability) is discussed in the Annexure-I. The hydrophobicity of any surface is determined by the contact angle >90°. The measured contact angle on most of the PP mask surfaces is found to be ~125°, which means PP masks can be utilized to avoid the spread of virus. It is important to note that household makeshift masks are often manufactured using cotton cloth/fabric, but the cotton material has been found to be hydrophilic and may not be suitable for making facemasks under prevalent conditions of the pandemic as the virus may travel through water droplets. In addition, the reusability of mask PP material is better compared to the cotton facemasks. The details are provided in Annexure-I.

Apart from wettability and reusability, the effective pore size of the facemask's surface determines the penetration of droplets released during coughing and sneezing. The pore size can be analyzed using a field-emission scanning electron microscope (FESEM) as described in Annexure-I. Often, an increase in the pore size due to insertion of a needle comes under question. Therefore, a study was carried out (details are provided in Annexure-I) on the PP material, and no evidence of pore size enhancement in the stitched region was observed.

For marketing purposes, bacterial filtration efficiency (BFE) as per the *ASTM standard F2101* should be studied. Furthermore, the particulate filter efficiency (PFE) tests as per standard ASTM F2299 must be carried out as a quality indicator for the manufactured facemasks. A study on these efficiencies was carried out, and details are provided in Annexure-I. The test reports clearly illustrate high efficiency of facemasks, with the bacterial filtration efficiency as high as 99.9% and particulate filtration efficiency as high as 95.46% along with good breathability (measured as pressure loss using the MS 36954C standard) and splash resistance (as per ASTM 1862) against synthetic blood.

The facemasks can be sterilized (decontaminate masks from viruses as well as bacteria) using UV-C (Figure 2.3) treatment with a wavelength of 254 nm. As shown in Figure 2.3, a number of UV-C lights have been fixed to provide appropriate dosage of UV-C during the manufacturing process. However, during the whole process, one must avoid direct exposure to UV-C light. Finally, the sterilized masks must be properly sealed and packed to maintain hygiene. This kind of know-how of facemask manufacturing is beneficial to the rural/small communities in two ways: firstly, it will help in generating awareness among the members of the rural community, and secondly, distribution of the locally produced masks will provide an avenue for income. For experimentation, around 100,000 facemasks developed by 200+ job-seekers were provided to various organizations. The experiment was successful with 100% acceptance of masks by users and a reasonable income for the needy people.

2.1.3 Portable UV-C light boxes

In addition to the abovementioned developments, the microenterprises can develop a portable disinfection box [4, 5] for small household articles like mobile phones, key rings, eyeglasses, watches, Bluetooth earphones, iPods, etc. apart from facemasks. The portable mask disinfecting box of dimension 12 inch × 5 inch × 4 inch is made of stainless steel with the inner surface wrapped with aluminum foil to increase reflectivity (Figure 2.4). The UV box is equipped with a 11 W UV-C lamp for disinfection. There is a switch at the top to start the sanitization process and the box is fitted with

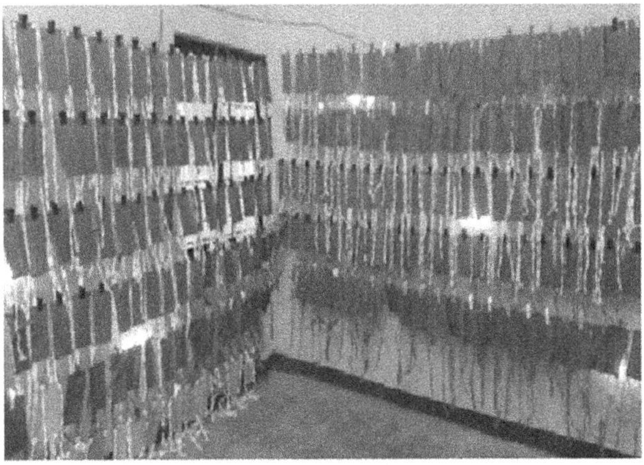

Figure 2.3 Developed facemasks being sterilized by UV-C light.

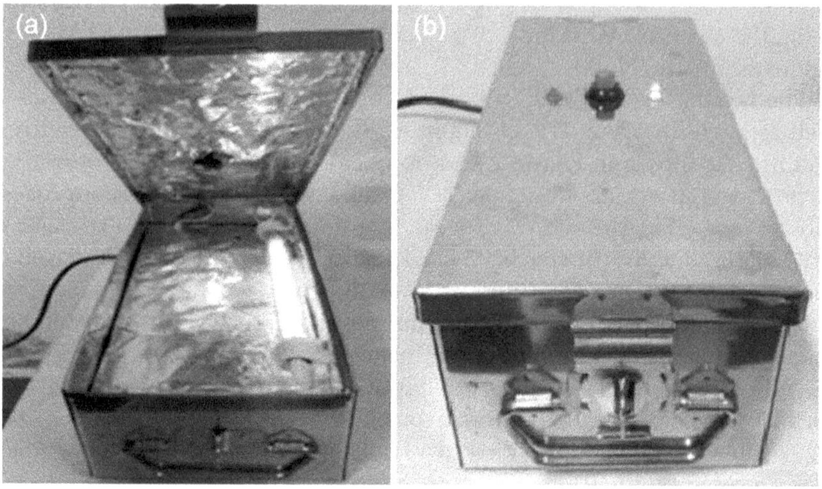

Figure 2.4 Portable UV-C light box.

a buzzer and an LED indicator that work during operation. To hang the mask properly, the UV box can be equipped with 2× 11 W UV-C lamps for disinfection. This box can sanitize any mask from both ends, as the mask can be hung using prefitted hooks on both sides of the wall.

2.2 SOAP AND DISPENSER

In communities where people are in constant contact with one another and surfaces covered with microorganisms, contaminated hands are the primary source of contact transmission (i.e., touching the mucosa of the mouth, nose, eyes) in spreading the virus across different surfaces. The virus can easily be inactivated and cleaned by soap solution. As per one estimate around three billion people lack hand sanitation facilities at home. To tackle this situation, daily liquid soap production capabilities are to be increased and the process needs to be easy to follow as per prescribed standards. To meet the needs of the society, the initiatives for the preparation of basic liquid soap and alcohol-based sanitizers in a cost-effective manner are required so that the products can be made affordable for the masses. To increase productivity, a process mechanization to meet the rising demand of soaps is described.

2.2.1 Basic liquid soap (BLS)

Soap making requires saponification of oil with appropriate proportions of caustic potash solution. The soap solution thus formed is mixed with a foaming agent, a moisturizing agent, appropriate color and essential oil for fragrance. The pH level of the soap solution is adjusted with a neutralizing agent until it reaches a desirable level. The complete process of soap making can be mechanized and a small plant can be fabricated so that large quantities of palm oil and caustic potash can be mixed with other important ingredients (sodium laureth sulfate (SLS), glycerine, boric acid, essential oil, color and distilled water) to produce soap in ample quantity on a daily basis [6]. The idea behind soap making is to provide hands-on training to the non-government organizations (NGOs) and self-help groups (SHGs) for downstream knowledge generation so that they can easily prepare soap for fighting the pandemic [6], as washing hands with soap and water is considered the best way to remove any enveloped virus from the hands. There are two different arguments on the usage of SLS. Some percentage of population experience skin irritation after exposure to SLS, which is time and dose dependent. To be on the safer side, SLS concentrations should not exceed 1%.

One major question arises, why soap and how is it effective? As the genetic material of the coronavirus is encased in a lipid envelope, to kill/inactivate the virus, there is a need to destroy the lipid envelope. Soaps can break the lipid envelope easily. At a nanometer level (shown in Figure 2.5), the structure of soap molecules is composed of water-loving (hydrophilic) heads and oil-loving (oleophilic) tails. During interaction between the coronavirus and soap tails, the long oleophilic tail of soap inserts itself into the envelope and breaks the lipid envelope of the virus. The tail also overpowers the bond that binds the RNA and thus dissolves the virus into its components, which can be easily removed by water [7]. Often the virus has been detected in human feces; therefore, washing hands with soap-water is needed to kill coronaviruses [8]. The process layout for mechanized production of liquid soap is given in Figure 2.6. This process plant is easy to make as it mainly contains pans/containers for oil, caustic potash, foaming

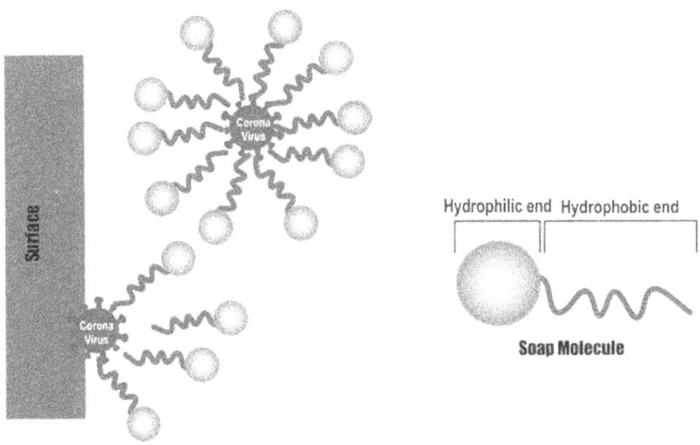

Figure 2.5 Action of soap molecules when used with water.

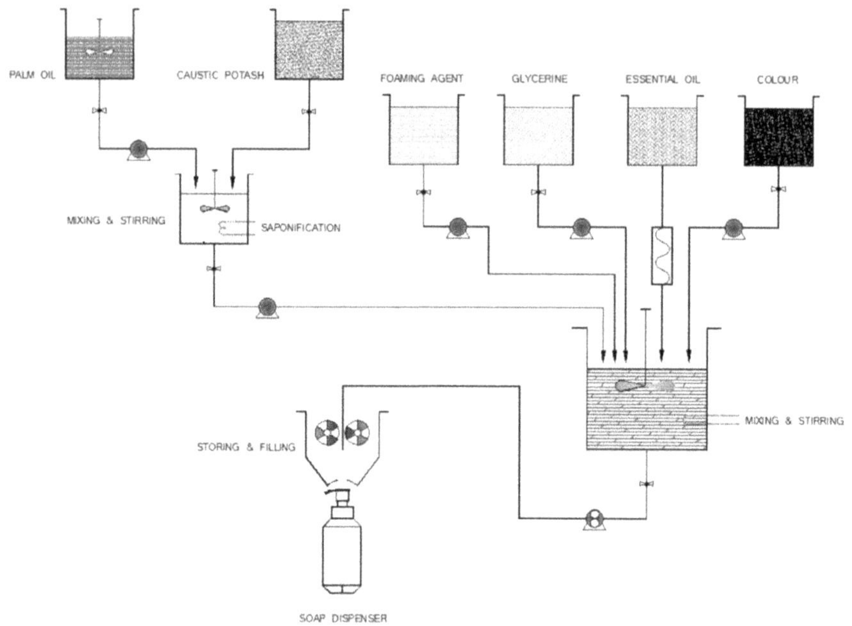

Figure 2.6 Process layout for mechanized production of liquid soap.

agents, glycerine, essential fragrance, color, motorized stirrers, control valves and filing devices.

2.2.2 Touch free soap dispensers

One of the most common practices for hand hygiene is soap-based hand cleansing. There is a need for a portable system to provide soap as well as water from the same outlet with a time gap of 20/30 seconds between soap and water to compel the user to rub hands for the essential time span as per standard sanitation guidelines. To cater to this requirement, a touch free soap-cum-water dispensing system [9], which utilizes a proximity sensor to activate the contactless delivery of soap/water, can be developed. Important features of this system (Figure 2.7) are:

- Soap and water dispensers with independent IR sensors (for soap and water).
- Portable soap dispensers using single IR sensors.
- Smart "tap" solutions for dispensing soap and water.
- Small size motorized pump.

A new system utilizing only one sensor and one tap is described in the next heading.

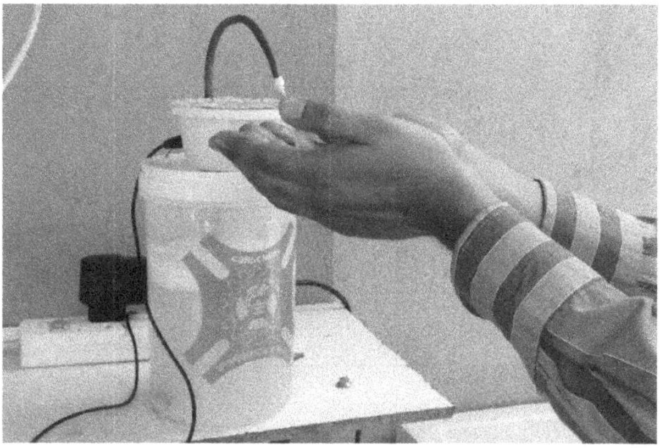

Figure 2.7 Developed touch free soap dispenser.

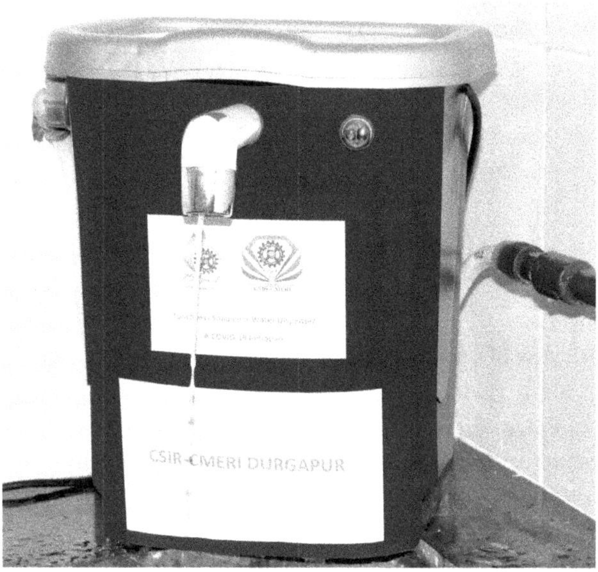

Figure 2.8 Touch free soap-cum-water dispensing system.

2.2.3 Portable touch free soap-cum-water dispensing system

Figure 2.8 displays the portable touch free soap-cum-water dispensing system [10, 11] utilizing a single sensor. It is worth noticing that there is a single tap dispenser for soap as well as water and it requires only one IR

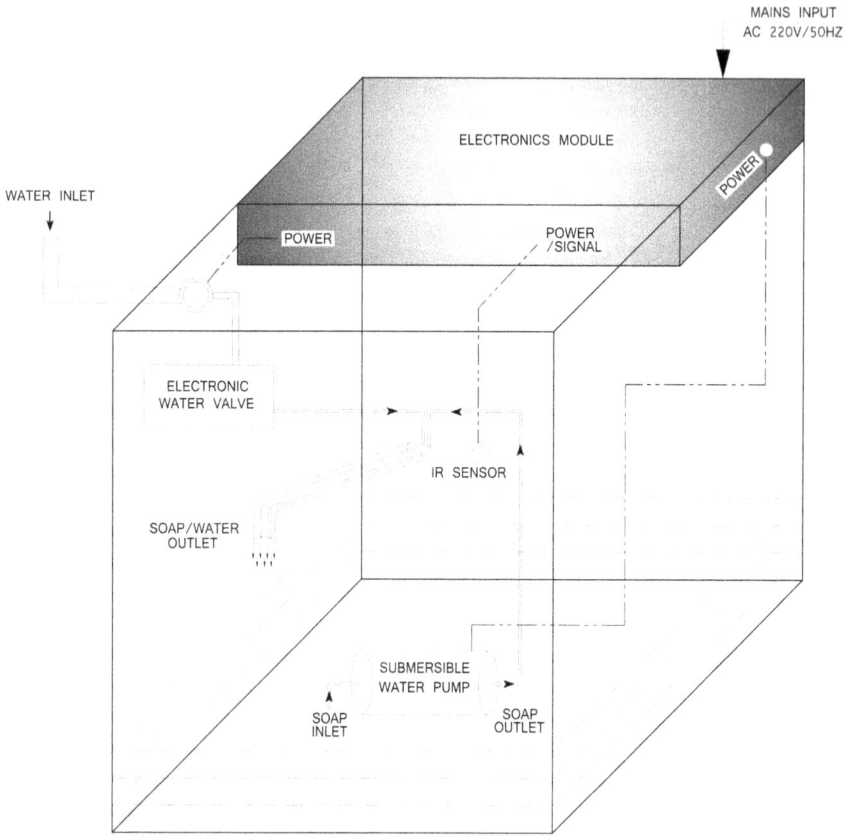

Figure 2.9 Block view of a soap dispensing system.

sensor. An open up view of the portable soap-cum-water dispensing system is represented in Figure 2.9. The operational procedure of the portable soap-cum-water dispensing system is given in Figure 2.10.

2.2.4 Portable touch free soap-cum-water dispensing system – compact version

Utility of the portable touch free soap-cum-water dispensing system [12] can be increased by making the system compact and by using a 12 V DC line for powering the electronic circuit. This kind of system will work on a small chargeable battery and will remain functional even in case of power failure. Figure 2.11 shows the developed portable touch free soap-cum-water dispensing system – a compact version. The few additional novelties of this system are:

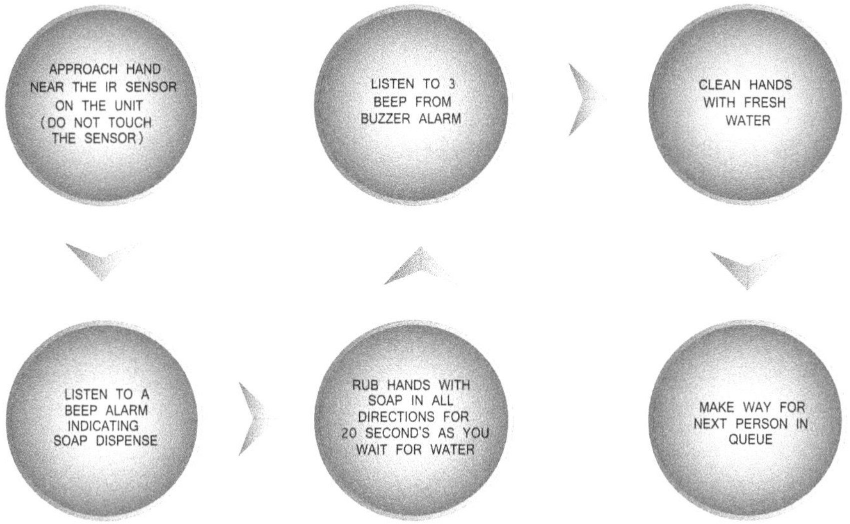
APPROACH HAND NEAR THE IR SENSOR ON THE UNIT (DO NOT TOUCH THE SENSOR)
LISTEN TO 3 BEEP FROM BUZZER ALARM
CLEAN HANDS WITH FRESH WATER
LISTEN TO A BEEP ALARM INDICATING SOAP DISPENSE
RUB HANDS WITH SOAP IN ALL DIRECTIONS FOR 20 SECOND'S AS YOU WAIT FOR WATER
MAKE WAY FOR NEXT PERSON IN QUEUE

Figure 2.10 Schematic of operational procedure of the portable soap-cum-water dispensing system.

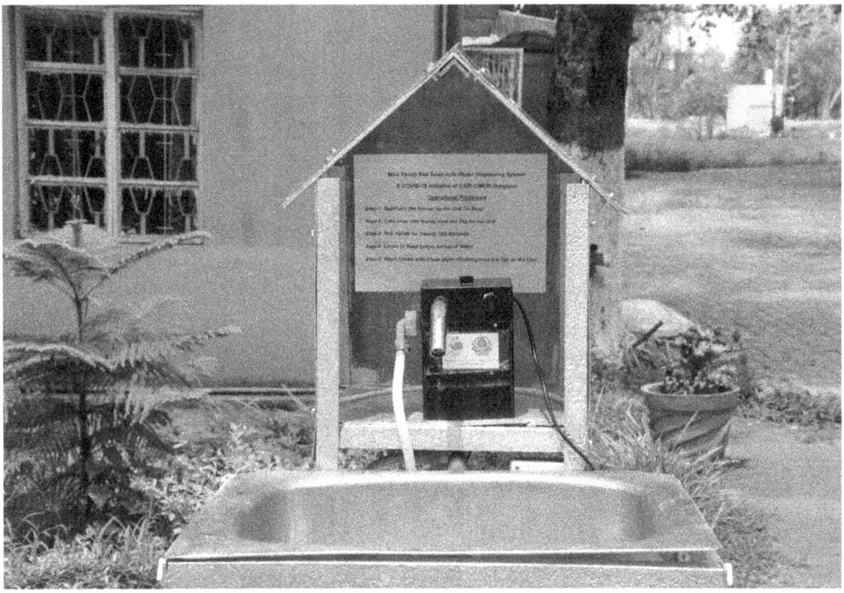

Figure 2.11 Developed portable touch free soap-cum-water dispensing system – compact version.

- Two variants: (1) table top and (2) wall mount.
- Material used: (1) acrylic (more attractive) and (2) powder-coated steel (more durable).

2.3 SANITIZER AND DISPENSER

Sanitizers can be classified as: alcohol-based and non-alcohol-based (i.e., benzalkonium chloride) sanitizers. Benzalkonium chloride (non-alcohol-based disinfectant) is preferred for clinical, food line, and domestic household biocides to inhibit growth of microorganisms. The sanitizers can quickly reduce the number of microbes through denaturing of enveloped layers but cannot remove the denatured cell walls and viral genomes from the hand. These kinds of sanitizers are less effective against "non-enveloped viruses" and "hands soiled with any dirt or grease".

2.3.1 Alcohol-based hand sanitizer

There are two types of alcohol-based hand sanitizers: (a) liquid hand sanitizer and (b) gel hand sanitizer. Ethyl/isopropyl alcohol is the main active ingredient in both the cases. These alcohols are rapidly bactericidal (kill bacteria and viruses) but do not destroy bacterial spores. Alcohols dissolve the protective lipid envelope of viruses, thus inactivating the viruses. In addition, alcohols present in hand sanitizers tend to change shape or destroy the spikes (that help the virus to bind to the receptor on the host cell surface and fuse their envelope with the cell) protruding from the lipid envelope. The US Food and Drug Administration (FDA) recommends the use of 60–95% ethanol or IPA in hand sanitizers to achieve better efficacy. The IPA-based liquid hand sanitizer process is described in the schematic diagram (Figure 2.12). The mode of action of hand sanitizer against virus and bacteria is represented in Figure 2.13. The digital images of the IPA-based liquid hand sanitizer bottles of different volumes are given in Figure 2.14. Often glycerine is added in the hand sanitizer to act as a moisturizer and to protect the skin from dryness. The presence of glycerine may increase the chances of bacterial growth; hydrogen peroxide is added to counter it.

2.4 DISINFECTION WALKWAY

Disinfectants, chemicals that destroy harmful pathogens/microorganisms, are recommended for cleaning and disinfecting surfaces to minimize spread of the pandemic virus. Disinfection walkways are passageways that spray disinfectant-mixed water on clothes/shoes of a human body to remove/deactivate/kill the pandemic-spreading virus. There is some difference in opinion about the existence and spread of virus through shoes and clothes.

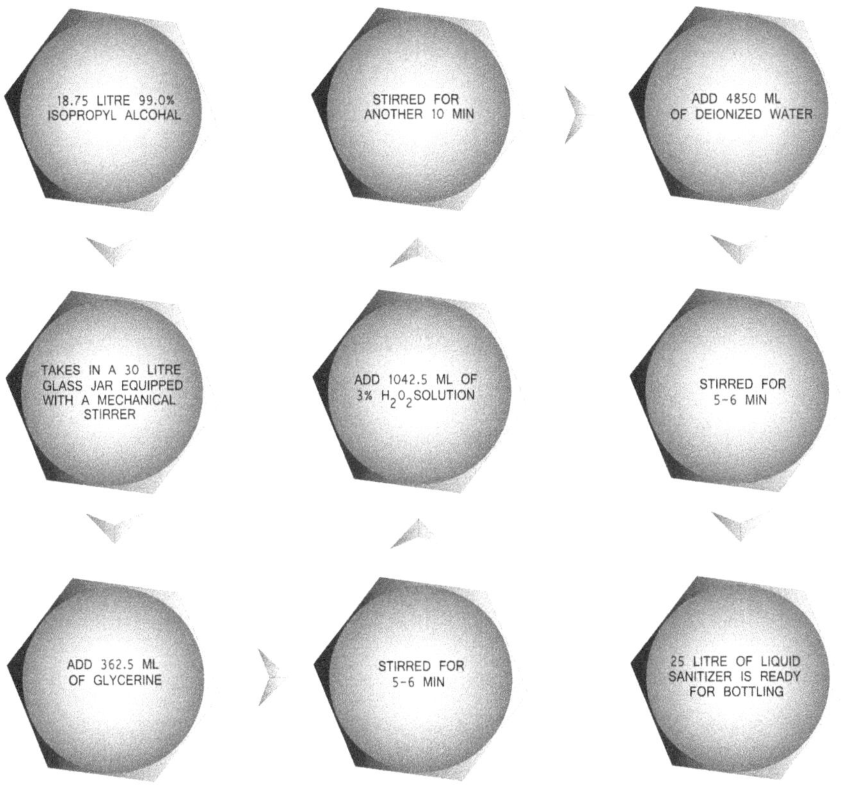

Figure 2.12 Schematic of preparation of 25 liters of IPA-based liquid.

One CDC report indicates the presence of COVID virus on clothes but with low survival probability. Other reports suggest that people, especially medical staff on the front lines could inadvertently be spreading the virus from its source, recommending stringent disinfecting measures [13]. To handle such risks, a disinfection walkway needs to be deployed at isolation/quarantine facilities, various entry points, medical centers, shopping malls, etc. The said disinfection walkways are available in two variants: hydraulic and pneumatic.

2.4.1 Hydraulic variant disinfection walkway

The "hydraulic variant disinfection walkway" is a spraying system designed for sanitizing every individual before entering into the main entrance gates of offices, hospitals, market premises [14], shopping complexes, housing societies, apartments, railway stations, etc., where movement of a large number of people occurs and there is more chance of spreading infections. The details on the design and construction of the system can be found in Annexure-I.

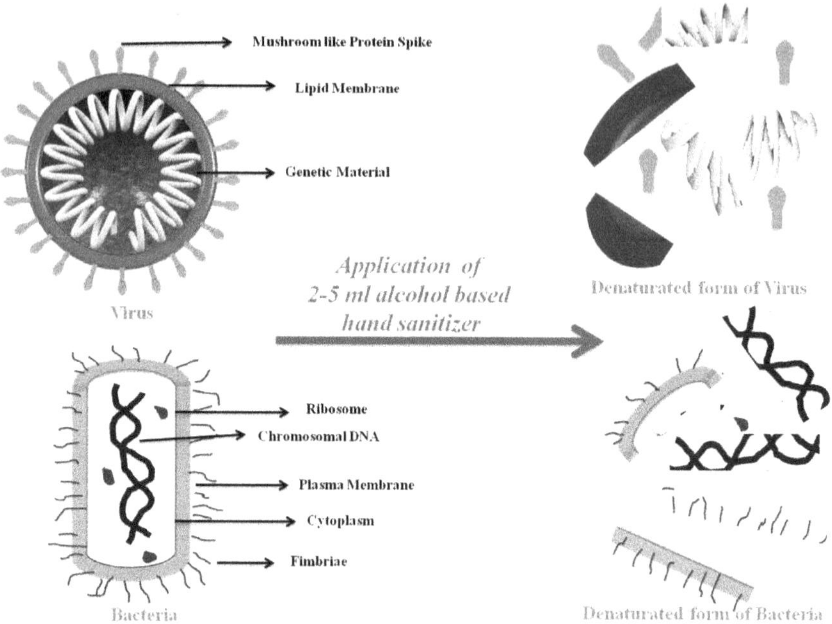

Figure 2.13 Mode of action of hand sanitizer against virus and bacteria.

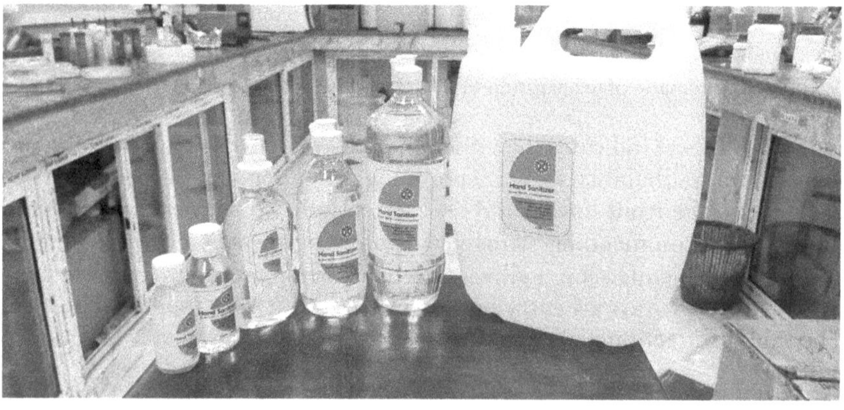

Figure 2.14 Digital images of the IPA-based liquid hand sanitizer bottles of different volumes.

2.4.2 Pneumatic variant disinfection walkway

The pneumatic disinfection walkway, comprising a housing walkway, one proximity sensor to detect entrance of a person, compressor and pneumatic pipelines, two water storage tanks, two different disinfecting chemicals and spray nozzles, can be considered as one of the most comprehensive disinfectant delivery systems [15]. The unit shall be installed at entry points of critical locations with a considerable amount of footfall and medical centers. The details on the design, construction and operation of the system can be found in Annexure-I.

2.5 DISINFECTANT SPRAYER

In spite of the trinity of practice of physical distancing, use of personal protective equipment and hand sanitization, pandemic virus may spread. To contain the virus, solutions of cleaning and disinfection of commonly touched (i.e., handrails, light/lift/road-crossing buttons, chair–tables, doorknobs, phones, keyboards, toilet faucets) surfaces in workplace/societies/school/marketplaces, etc. are required. The virus spreads mainly in two ways: the first way of virus spread is via airborne droplets (>5 μm) and aerosols (smaller than 5 μm). The droplets are expelled into the air through a cough or sneeze and quickly settle down to the ground [16] or another surface. Aerosols being smaller in size remain in air for a longer time (finally getting dispersed by drying out).

The second way of pandemic spread is via frequently touched surfaces having few settled droplets encapsulating the virus. Different types of materials, recommended by CDC and WHO, can be used as disinfectant spray, depending on types of objects:

- Frequently touched surfaces: Chlorine-containing disinfectants (1000 mg/l), chlorine dioxide (500 mg/l), 75% alcohol.
- Hands: Alcohol-based disinfectants, hydrogen peroxide.
- Skin: Iodine-based disinfectants, hydrogen peroxide, quaternary ammonium salt, benzalkonium chloride, 2% triclosan.

To spray the disinfectant, mechanical devices are required, which are explained in the following subsections.

2.5.1 Tractor-mounted road sanitizing unit

The tractor-mounted road sanitizing unit is designed for road sanitization [17, 18]. This unit utilizes a tractor and a normal water tank. A high pressure (350 PSI max) pump mounted on the designed base plate with a support structure fixed with the tractor is controlled by the power takeoff (PTO) of the tractor through a belt pulley arrangement, so the need for additional power source is eliminated. A tractor-mounted road sanitizer has been shown in Figure 2.15, and the schematic diagram of the sanitizing unit is provided in Figure 2.16. It is worth noting that spraying disinfectant into the air may reduce the amount of virus suspended as aerosols. However, this may be effective for a limited time depending upon the environmental (i.e., sunshine, dust particles) conditions. More details on the design, construction and operation of the unit can be found in Annexure-I.

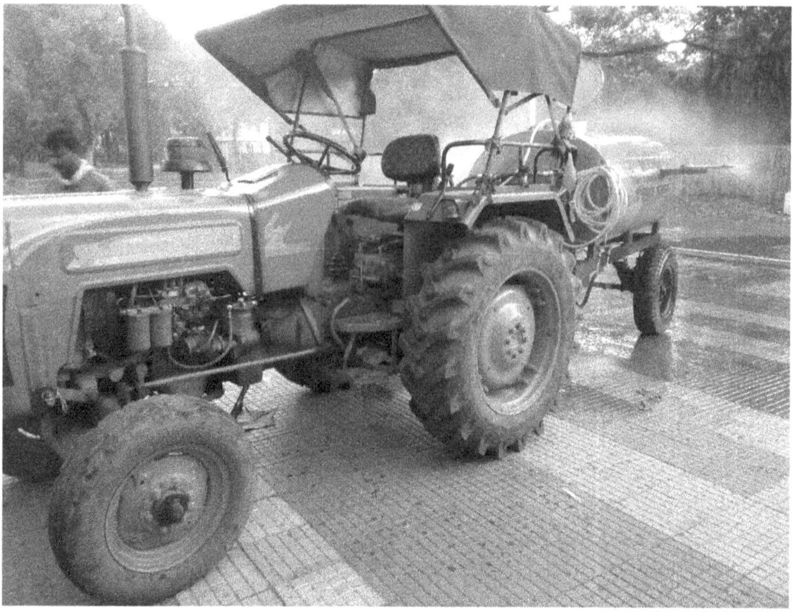

Figure 2.15 Developed tractor-mounted road sanitizer.

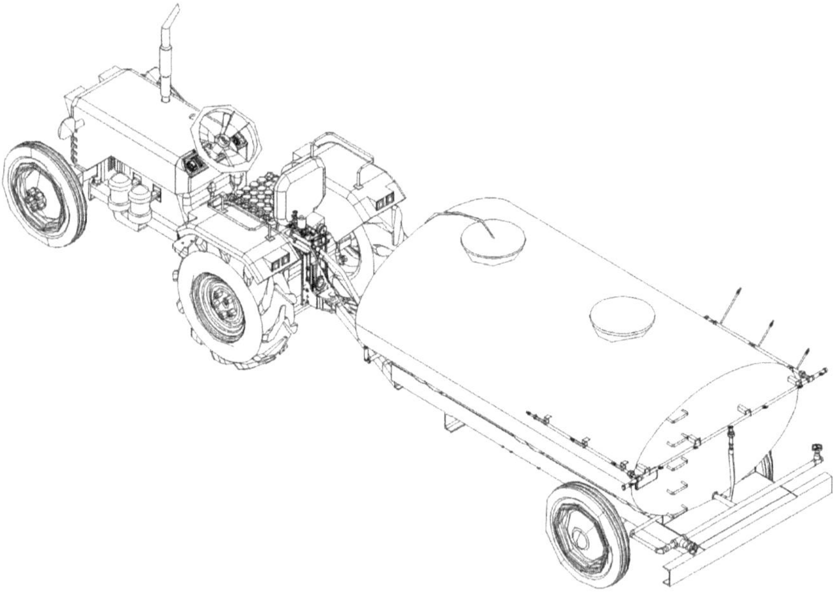

Figure 2.16 Schematic diagram of a tractor-mounted road sanitizing unit.

2.5.2 Pneumatically operated mobile indoor disinfection (POMID) unit

The POMID unit [19] may be used for removal, deactivation or killing of pathogenic microorganisms present inside a closed chamber like rooms, halls, building corridors using water/other liquids mixed with chemical disinfectants. Compressed air is used to form mist/jet spray of liquid disinfectants to sanitize the indoor area. This unit is mounted on a four-wheel trolley to make it movable. The system comprises a pneumatic compressor system, two storage tanks for two different disinfectants and spray systems with a mopping facility. More details on the design features and operation of the unit can be found in Annexure-I.

2.5.3 Battery powered disinfectant sprayer (BPDS)

This disinfectant unit may be used for the deactivating or killing of pathogenic microorganisms present on the surfaces/environment by spraying water-soluble chemical disinfection mist [20]. The unit is designed for the ease of retrofitting on a standard wheelchair used in hospitals. The sprayer is equipped with a mopping feature which also enables the mopping of the floors and soaking the spread chemicals from the floor. Figure 2.17

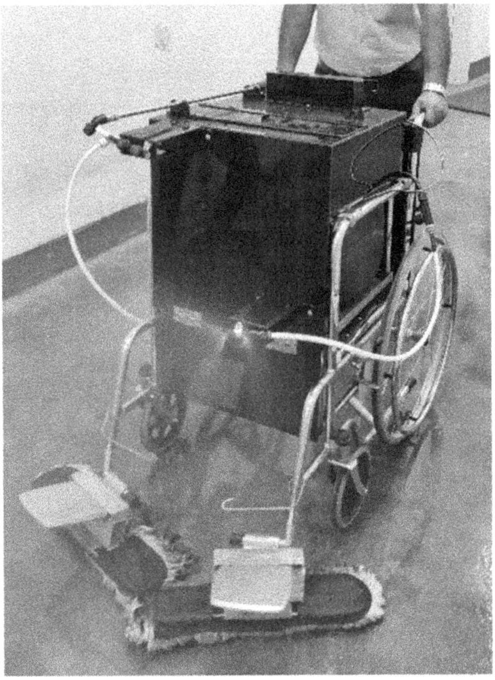

Figure 2.17 Developed battery powered disinfectant sprayer.

shows the developed BPDS. The working principle of the BPDS is depicted in Figure 2.18, and the evolution of the disinfectant sprayer system is presented in Figure 2.19.

Owing to a number of features in the BPDS, the system can be used for following applications:

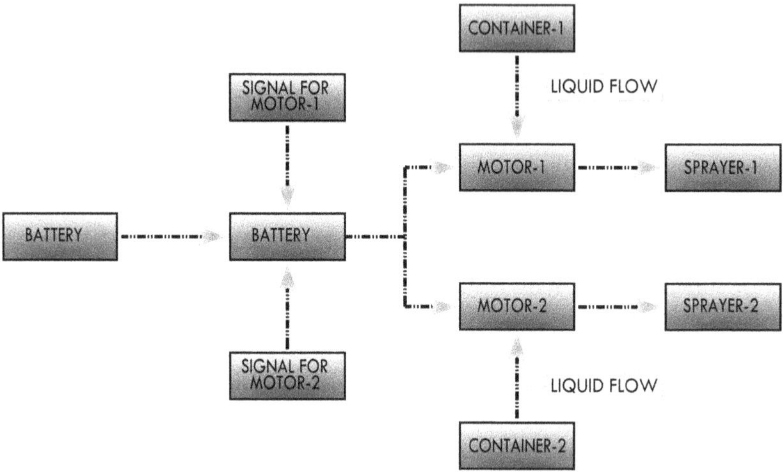

Figure 2.18 Working principle of the BPDS.

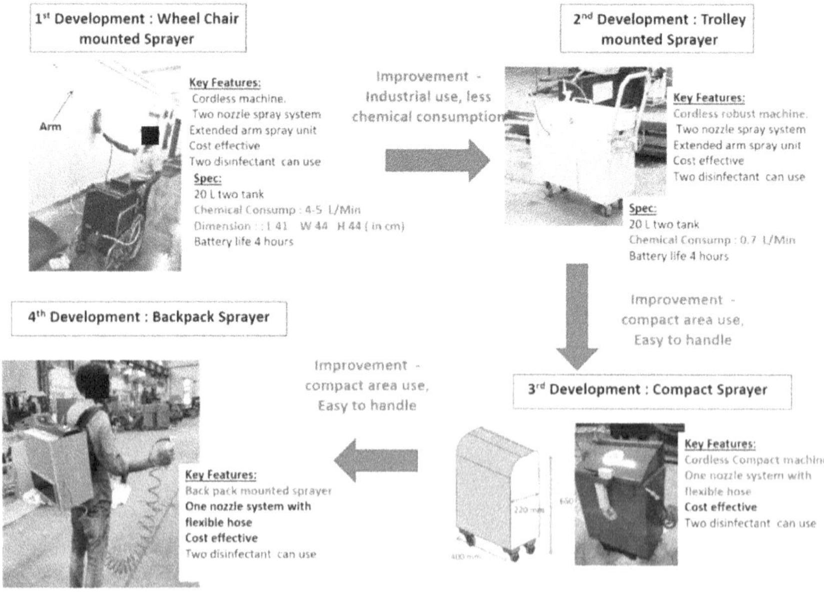

Figure 2.19 Evolution of the disinfectant sprayer system.

- Cleaning of office rooms on an everyday basis. Dirty contact surfaces can be cleaned with soap and water prior to disinfection.
- All contact surfaces of entrance lobbies, corridors, staircases, escalators, elevators, call buttons, security guard booths, intercom systems, printers/scanners, table tops, chair handles, pens, diary, keyboards, mouse, mouse pad, tea/coffee dispensing machines, door handles, security locks, keys, toilet floor, sink, taps and fittings, etc., and 70% alcohol can be used where the use of other disinfectants are unsuitable.
- Outdoor areas such as bus stops, railway platforms, parks, etc.

2.6 MEDICAL HELP

There is a possibility of the pandemic virus affecting the lungs of an individual by multiplying the growth rate within the respiratory system and reducing the oxygen supply to the lungs. These patients often need supplemental oxygen for faster recovery from the infection. In general, concentrated oxygen is delivered to the patient such that their oxygen saturation stabilizes and is maintained within normal ranges. To address the future viability of oxygen requirement, it is to be noted that oxygen therapy will be relevant even in the days to come, since it is used as a non-invasive therapy for faster wound healing, cell repair and self-healing of organs. In addition, there is tremendous potential for applications in the domains of high-altitude defense as well as in places with high altitude having significant tourist footfalls where it can be used as oxygen rejuvenation hubs for fatigued tourists. Oxygen should be treated as an essential utility, as vital as electricity or water [21].

2.6.1 Oxygen enrichment unit

Easiest way to provide oxygen therapy is to concentrate oxygen, by separating the nitrogen from air using porous zeolite adsorbents. Due to the large microporous surface area inside the zeolite adsorbents, nitrogen from atmospheric air can be adsorbed under pressure higher than the atmosphere, and as an output, a stream of enriched oxygen can be achieved. The adsorbent can be regenerated by decreasing the pressure to release the adsorbed nitrogen. In this way, a continuous oxygen stream supply can be generated to assist an individual and increase the fraction of inspired oxygen. One of such oxygen enrichment units (OEUs), based on the pressure swing adsorption (PSA) technique is illustrated in Figure 2.20. This oxygen enrichment unit is also suitable for simultaneous use by multiple patients, as shown in Figure 2.21. This decentralized OEU is advantageous as it costs less. Due to the remote location of the compressor, it operates silently, occupies less space and can be installed at the bedside with control on the FiO_2 ratio. Such a decentralized OEU system with a bedside regulator can regulate flow with an accuracy of 0.5 LPM and finds its use in "high flow oxygen

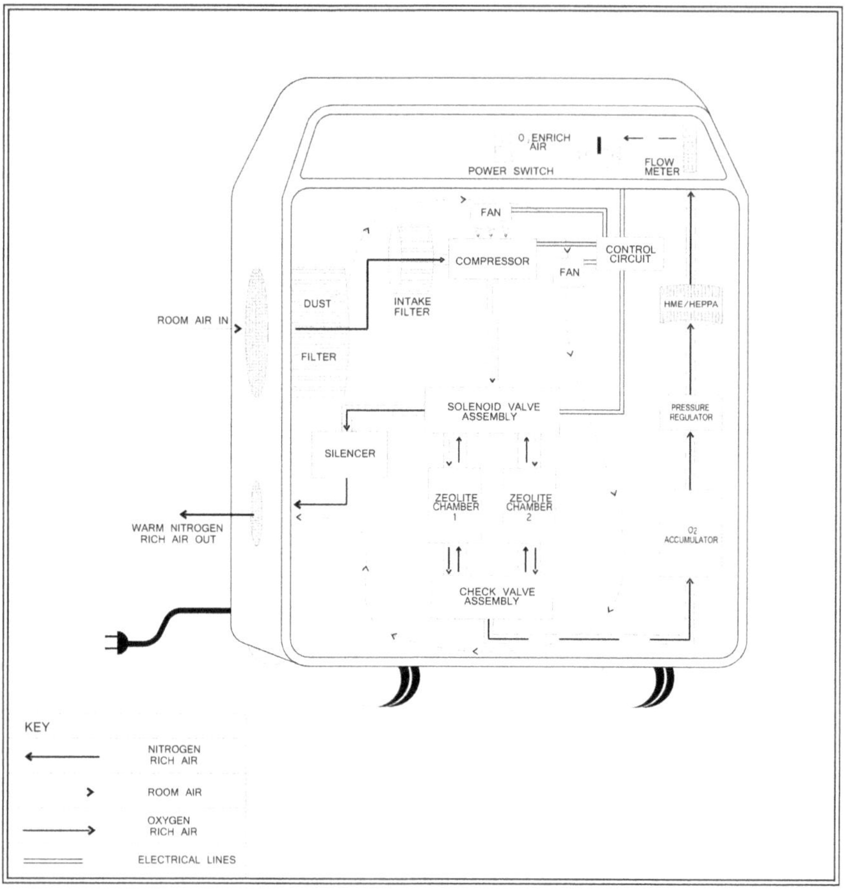

Figure 2.20 Schematic diagram of oxygen enrichment unit.

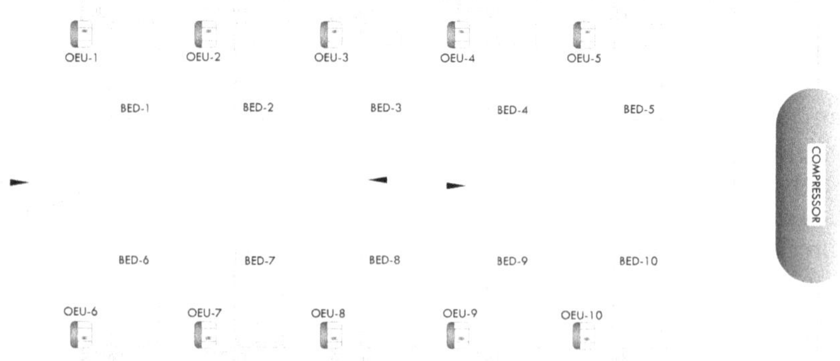

Figure 2.21 The CSIR-CMERI OEU for simultaneous supply of oxygen to multiple patients.

therapy", which is proven to be a better method in treatment and management of COVID-19 patients.

2.6.2 Mechanical ventilator

Pandemic diseases may create respiratory problems and damage the respiratory system causing (1) shortage of O_2 and accumulation of CO_2; (2) disruption of biochemical activities within the human body; (3) lack of oxygen reducing life of tissues and leading to failure of organs and finally increasing chances of patient death. In such cases, the medical ventilator externally maintains the respiratory system to keep the patient alive. For ease of understanding, the ventilator and its functions have been presented graphically in Figure 2.22. It is necessary to understand that a mechanical

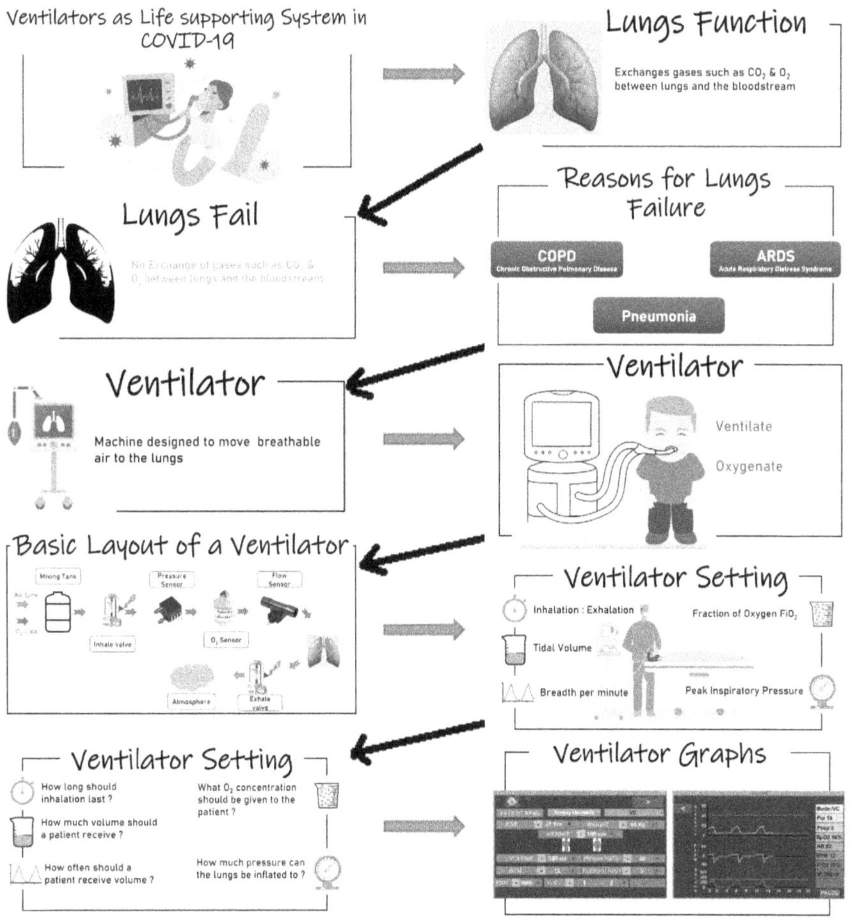

Figure 2.22 Graphic representation of a ventilator and its functions.

ventilator buys time for the patient so that sufferer responds to various medical treatments, but it is not a permanent solution. Often adverse effects of mechanical ventilation occur, as the required setting for every patient is different, which is very difficult to judge at the beginning of treatment. Even more difficult is various settings of the ventilator for the same patient during sleeping, during lying down and during some activity. Due to inappropriate volume/pressure settings of the ventilator lung damage increases, this further deteriorates the patient's health. Therefore, mechanical ventilation should be a last resort, particularly during a pandemic when medical experts will not be able to carefully manage all the parameters.

During pandemics, hospitals face severe shortages in ICU beds with oxygen and mechanical ventilators [22], which are essentially required for the patients who are critically ill. In the absence of a proper screening mechanism, hospitals generally allot these ICU beds to patients who have a falling SpO_2 (below 85%) on a first come first serve basis to avoid any controversy. This results in a situation where a patient who really needs these resources is denied admission owing to unavailability of ICU beds. These situations may force the authorities to develop makeshift quarantine/isolation wards for the affected patients, causing emergency requirements of cost-effective ventilators. These mechanical ventilators, in combination with appropriate medications and support of nursing/medical support staff, become a deciding factor between life and death of a critical patient. As per the FDA guidelines, any ICU ventilator should have "declaration of conformity" with the following standards:

1. IEC 60601-1: 2012: Medical electrical equipment – part 1: general requirements for basic safety and essential performance.
2. IEC 60601-1-2: 2014: Medical electrical equipment part 1-2: general requirements for basic safety and essential performance – collateral standard: electromagnetic disturbances – requirements and tests.
3. ISO 80601-2-12:2020: Medical electrical equipment – Part 2-12: particular requirements for basic safety and essential performance of critical care ventilators.

Some studies reveal that most of the patients may be cured through oxygen therapy alone without needing ventilation. This means an intermediate affordable system should be developed, which can act as an oxygen enrichment unit and continuously monitor SpO_2. If even after providing the needed oxygen, the SpO_2 level does not rise above 90%, then ventilator mode should be switched on. In the worst case, if an affordable ventilator does not respond to the patient's condition, then only the patient may be shifted to the full-fledged ventilator of the ICU. Based on this thinking, an advanced multifunctional ventilator with an integrated oxygen enrichment unit capable of providing normal as well as nasal high flow (NHF) oxygen therapies can be developed. The unit is capable of enriching oxygen and supplying to the patient and has an inbuilt SpO_2 measuring sensor that displays the patient data in real time. This innovation has been tuned to perform all the tasks as highlighted in Figure 2.23.

The specifications of the advanced multifunctional ventilator with an integrated oxygen enrichment unit are:

Specifications:

A microcontroller along with pressure and flow sensors in a closed loop:

- Continuously monitors and displays pressure, volume and flow with time in the monitor.
- Parameters can be set on the fly through the GUI-like tidal volume, BPM, inspiratory:expiratory (I:E) ratio, PEEP and PIP.
- Alarms for different set limits.

Mechanical fail-safe valve opens at 80 cm H_2O if there is electrical/electronic failure

PIP:	40–70 cm H_2O adjustable in steps of 5 cm H_2O
PEEP:	5–20 cm H_2O adjustable in steps of 5 cm H_2O
Inspiratory:expiratory ratio (I:E):	1:1–1:3 (adjustable)
Respiratory rate (BPM):	10–30 breaths per minute in increments of 2
Tidal volume:	350 mL–650 mL in steps of 50 ml

Modes available ("volume assist/control"):

- Volume control (VC) – continuous mandatory ventilation (CMV) for passive patients.
- Volume control (VC) – intermittent mandatory ventilation (IMV) for partially active patients

2.6.3 Hospital care assistive robotic devices

The increasing trend of infection of the health workers and doctors in pandemic situation need innovative solutions so that two-way audio-visual communication between the patient and the healthcare staff/doctors, opening and closing the of drawers for delivery of foods, medicines, etc. are carried out by the nursing staff sitting in remotely located booth outside the ward. To support their tireless efforts hospital care assistive robotic device (HCARD) [23] can be developed to ensure seamless contact-free communication and delivery of medical intervention between the healthcare personnel and the patients. HCARD, a guided vehicle, can follow predefined paths marked on the floor and reach various locations inside the ward. Apart from the guided mode, the robot can also be operated using a joystick. HCARD is equipped with an obstacle detection feature. All the drawers are fitted with UV lights to reduce hospital acquired infections. Using this robotic device, the healthcare personnel in hospitals can attend the patients

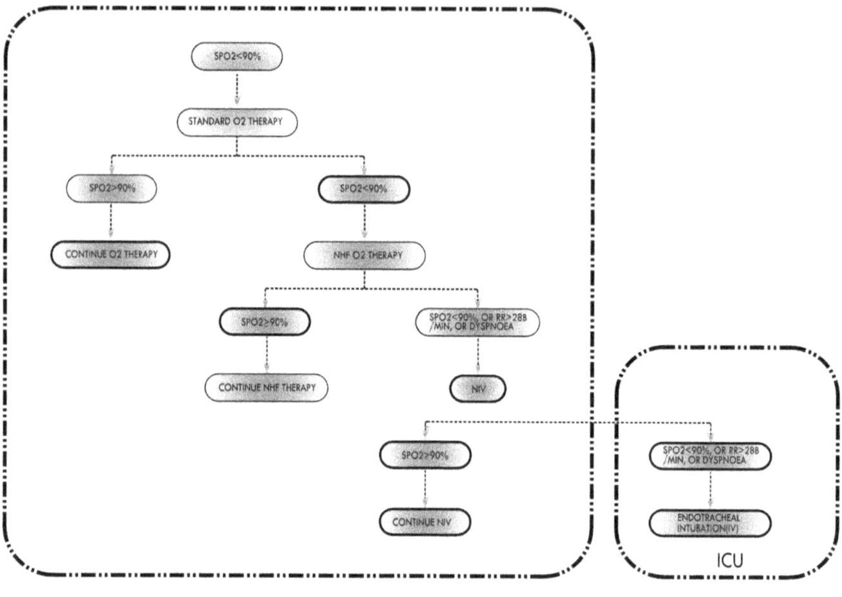

Figure 2.23 Schematic of advanced oxygen-based treatment.

maintaining physical distancing from them. Continuous (24×7) operation is possible with such a system owing to the manual swapping of batteries. An indicator constantly monitors the status of the residual charge of the battery pack and upon reaching the threshold limit an audible alarm is generated so that the batteries can be changed/charged. The image of the HCARD with technical specifications has been shown in Figure 2.24.

Apart from the HCARD, digital services can be initiated in the healthcare sectors to minimize the distance-based issues of health workers so that they spend more time on delivering essential healthcare services. The healthcare services can be availed by people whenever and wherever required. Thus, each recipient is reachable for follow-up for making the solutions sustainable.

2.7 HOSPITAL WASTE MANAGEMENT FACILITY

Waste generated during the diagnosis/treatment/immunization or waste created during production/testing of biological samples is termed as hospital waste. The medical waste may contain infectious plastic/metallic, hazardous and other biomedical wastes. Ideally appropriate segregation, transportation and safe disposal methods are required. The unscientific and improper disposal of hospital waste containing toxic and biohazardous contaminants trigger the chance of outbreak of the hazardous substance to

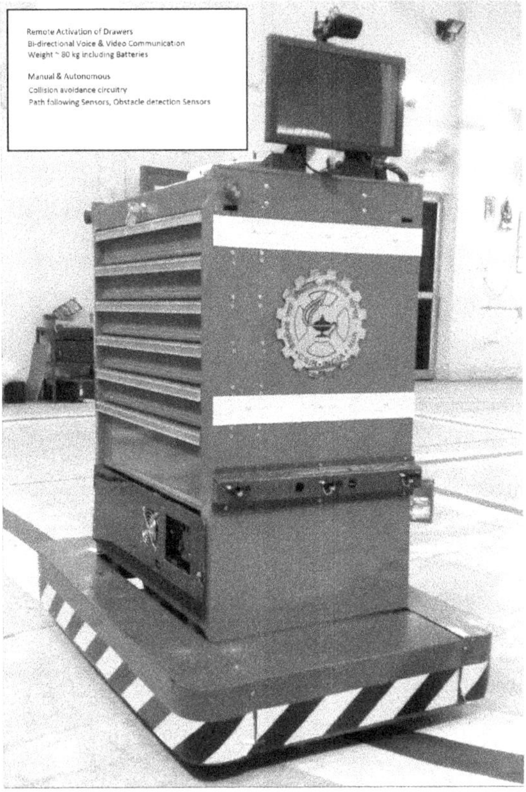
Remote Activation of Drawers
Bi-directional Voice & Video Communication
Weight ~ 80 kg including Batteries
Manual & Autonomous
Collision avoidance circuitry
Path following Sensors, Obstacle detection Sensors

Figure 2.24 Developed hospital care assistive robotic device with technical specifications.

the environment. Under this definition, all single use PPE (i.e., masks, face shields, gloves, head caps, aprons) and reusable PPE after their appropriate service should be discarded appropriately. In this regard, one of thermal degradation process, such as shown in Figure 2.25 is required. A plasma arc-driven technology comprising plasma electrodes for the generation of high temperature plasma (2000~3000°C), which results in complete decomposition and destruction of pathogens, is the latest best available method. Incineration, the most commonly used method may release toxic gases causing the spread of diseases. To generate a very high temperature (>2000°C) plasma torch is used.

The gas handling system and the secondary burning chamber must be designed to maintain toxic emission like total dioxin and furan emission, below the Central Pollution Control Board (CPCB) safe limit (<0.01 ng. TEQ/Nm^3). The schematic representations of a plasma-assisted hospital solid waste (HSW) disposal plant, a plasma arc-assisted 15 kg/h HSW disposal pilot plant and a 1 TPD hospital solid waste disposal plant have

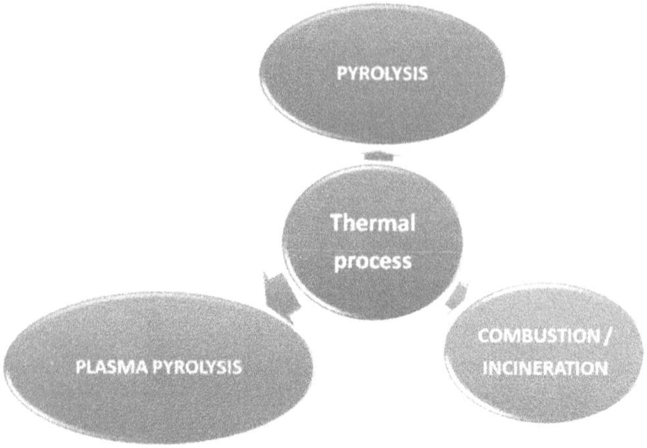

Figure 2.25 Thermal decomposition processes for medical waste.

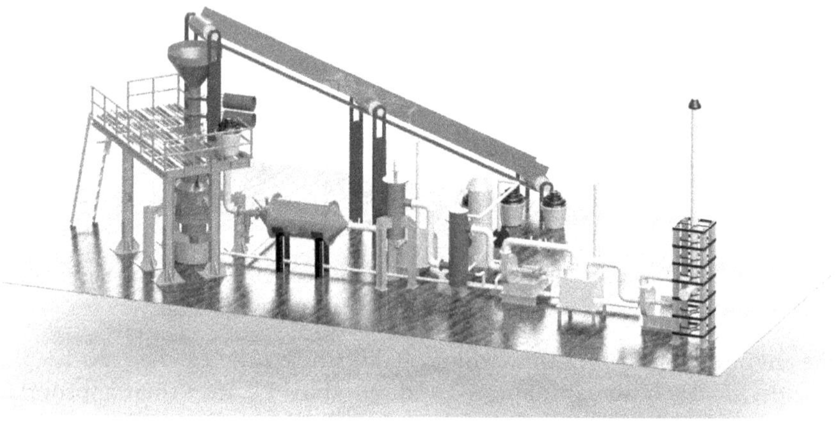

Figure 2.26 Schematic representation of a plasma-assisted hospital solid waste disposal plant.

been shown in Figures 2.26, 2.27 and 2.28, respectively. The preamble, novelty and deployment status of the systems are:

Preamble and novelty

- High temperature (~2000–3000°C) plasma arc-assisted eco-friendly disposal of HSW with high waste destruction efficiency (~85–90%) by mass and combustion efficiency (>99%).
- Level of toxin emission from the HSW treatment plant lies below the CPCB standard of toxic gas emission.

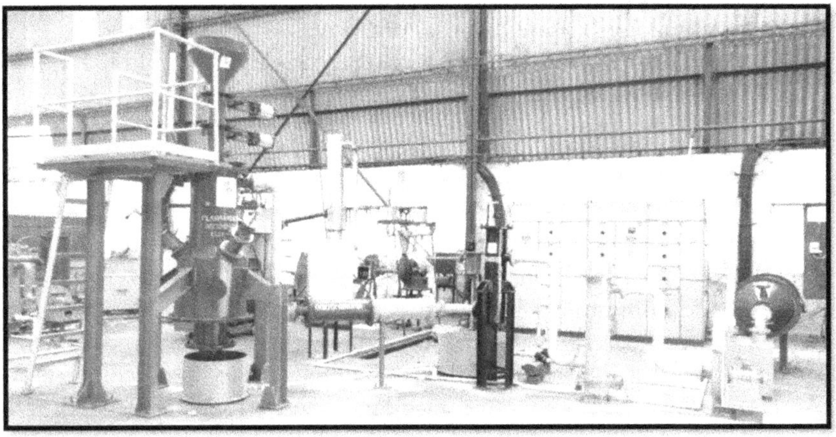

Figure 2.27 A plasma arc-assisted 15 kg/h hospital solid waste disposal pilot plant.

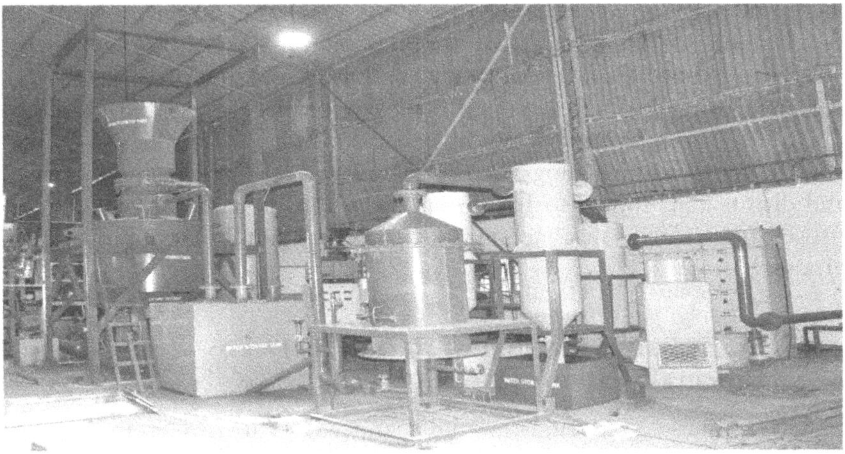

Figure 2.28 One TPD hospital solid waste disposal plant.

- Process routes of hospital waste are safe, hygienic, efficient, easy to control and in compliance with hospital waste management rules prescribed by the CPCB.
- Major system components include a plasma gasifier, a secondary chamber, an electrode and a gas cleaning unit comprising a catalytic converter, a scrubber, a booster drive and a chimney.

Deployment

- The developed technology is tested at a laboratory level with different controlling parameters. It is now ready for field deployment.

- Various healthcare organizations like hospitals, health centers can use this technology for safe disposal of HSW.
- Governments, NGOs can utilize this technology to build a commercially viable waste management facility.

2.8 COVID PROTECTION SYSTEM (COPS) FOR GATED COMMUNITY/COMPLEXES

Upon entering any gated community/complex, there is a high risk of infecting the entire community by an infected visitor. The security guards, entrusted with the responsibilities of temperature reading and sanitizer dispensing, are the most vulnerable individuals, since they come to the closest proximity of any visiting outsiders. Even a foot-pedaled sanitizer dispenser is very risky as it exposes a weak link to the spread of contamination through shoes to the community. There is also a high risk of contamination and spread in a gated community through visiting cars. Therefore, there is a need to automate all inspection and sanitization methods and develop appropriate software to remotely monitor and minimize the risk of human exposure to the pandemic. Based on this thinking, the COVID protection system (COPS), an artificial intelligence-augmented protective shield for any organization, can be developed. The COPS harnesses imaging, thermal scanning, upgraded nozzle design, sensor-based automation and disinfectant fogger to battle the virus transmission. The COPS consists of four-pronged mechanisms to enforce and handle entry management protocols.

2.8.1 Solar-based intelligent mask ATM-cum-thermal scanner (IntelliMAST)

Intelligent mask ATM-cum-thermal scanner (IntelliMAST), an AI-based intelligent machine identifies the person with or without a facemask. An automatic IR-based thermal scanning mechanism of IntelliMAST takes a person's body temperature for deciding whether they should get entry into the institution or not. The machine, in the first phase, detects the person coming in its proximity and checks forehead temperature using an IR-based thermal sensor. If the system finds the body temperature of the person higher than the permissible limit, it raises an audio-visual alarm, otherwise it enters into the second phase of the scanning process and the system takes photographs of the person using a built-in camera. Computer vision is used to identify the facial features of the person. The detected facial features are then fed to an AI engine equipped with a pretrained deep learning model (trained for classifying masked and non-masked faces with higher than 98% precision). Further details of this system are provided in Annexure-I.

2.8.2 Touchless faucet (TouF): washbasin-mounted contactless soap-cum-water dispensing unit

The touchless faucet (detailed in Annexure-I) can be very easily mounted by replacing the existing tap of any washbasin. This system dispenses water 30 seconds after dispensing soap in a touch free mechanism. When a person approaches the sensor on the basin-mounted touchless faucet, a predefined amount of soap (few milliliters) will be dispensed from the tap, momentarily. After rubbing hands for 30 seconds, clean water is dispensed from the same tap. The arrangement aims to reduce wastage of water and is suited for homes and offices. The system also works manually in case of a power failure. More details are listed in Annexure-I.

2.8.3 360° car flusher

The 360° car flusher [24] is developed for sanitization of cars, trucks, buses, etc. The sanitizing system can be used in long stretches of highways, vicinity of markets, shopping malls, office campuses as well as residential complexes, etc. The active sensor-based automatic power supply to a pump is used in this technology. Hence, no manual intervention is required to operate the pump. Figure 2.29 shows the developed 360° car flusher. More details on the component features and operational principles of the system can be found in Annexure-I.

2.8.4 Dry fogging shoe disinfector (DFSD)

Various studies suggest that virus spread occurs from the soles of shoes [13]. The shoe soles of medical staff act as virus carriers; therefore, disinfection

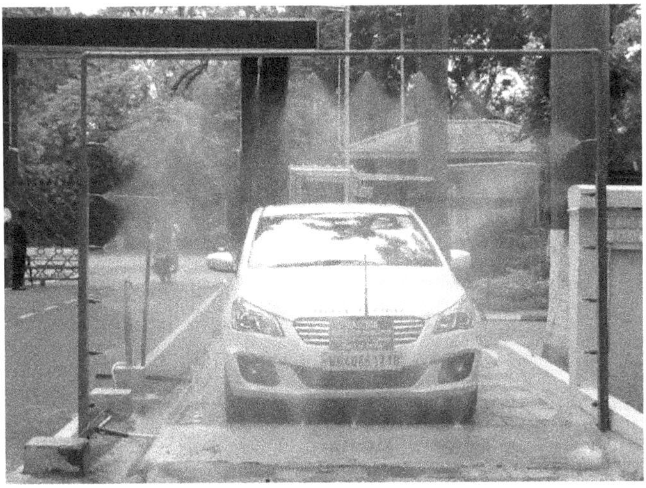

Figure 2.29 Developed 360° car flusher.

of shoe soles before walking out of hospital wards is recommended. The dry fogging shoe disinfector (DFSD) atomizes water-based disinfectants into very fine size (<10 micron) particles to ensure that the number of particles cluster around the pathogens stuck on the shoe sole and enables higher contact time of the disinfectant with the microorganisms present. The smaller size of the particles also guarantees minimum wetting of the surfaces and no damage of shoe leather/Rexine material. Details on the operation of the system can be found in Annexure-I.

2.9 CONCLUSIONS

During any pandemic, when the situation everywhere is at an emergency level, it is very important that a seamless flow of information, knowledge and technology among the various adjacent communities is provided to ensure that the pandemic is tackled comprehensively. Equipping the communities with the know-how and adequate skills would empower them to act in a decentralized and democratic manner and handle the ravages of the pandemic right from the grassroot level. This will also help in redirecting the course of the pandemic itself, as collectively the different communities will be able to steer the nation toward responsible handling of the pandemic. Since, there is always a risk of simultaneous explosion from the transmission, it is very important that there is a decentralized strategy ready for deployment as and when needed.

Government funds the projects to perform financial-risky research in national laboratories and academic institutions so that successful research outcomes are translated into commercial ventures, which would indirectly help in ensuring widespread application of the technologies for socioeconomic utilization. Consequently, this would also help in improving the employment and economic prospects of the people in the region. Collectively these communities, empowered by a robust technology backup will provide a veritable front for combating the ill-effects of the pandemic.

BIBLIOGRAPHY

1. Milton, DK., Fabian, MP., Cowling, BJ., Grantham, ML., McDevitt, JJ. Influenza Virus Aerosols in Human Exhaled Breath: Particle Size, Culturability, and Effect of Surgical Masks. *PLoS Pathog* 9(3): e1003205, 2013, https://doi.org/10.1371/journal.ppat.1003205
2. https://wwwnc.cdc.gov/eid/article/26/7/20-0885_article#share-nav, 2022
3. Poulami Roy, Partha Sarathi Pal, Nilrudra Mandal, Himadri Roy, and Harish Hirani. Process know-how to manufacture three layered hydrophobic surface mask along with UV-C sterilization process. Copyright Application, CMERI Ref. IPMG/Copyright/2020-21/159, 2020.

4. Imtiaz Alam, Partha Sarathi Pal, and Harish Hirani. Programmable logic and hardware interfacing circuit for a contactless and fully automatic UVC-254 disinfectant cabinet. Copyright Application, CMERI Ref. IPMG/Copyright/2020-21/169, 2020.
5. Saurav Halder, Kalyan Chatterjee, Nripen Chanda, Nilrudra Mandal, and Harish Hirani. Small UV disinfector box. Copyright Application, CMERI Ref. IPMG/Copyright/2020-21/170, 2020.
6. https://www.thehindu.com/sci-tech/science/how-does-soap-use-help-in-tackling-covid-19/article31070630.ece, 2022
7. https://www.nationalgeographic.com/science/2020/03/why-soap-preferable-bleach-fight-against-coronavirus/, 2022
8. https://theprint.in/health/this-is-what-makes-the-humble-soap-our-best-bet-against-coronavirus/380799/, 2022
9. Jyotirmoy Karmakar, Siva Ram Krishna Vadali, Manoj Kumar Biswal, Sandeep Jain, and Harish Hirani. Design of a single sensor and single outlet based soap and water dispensing system. Design Registration, CSIR Ref. 7/Design/2020, 2020.
10. Jnanendra Prasad Maji, Imtiaz Alam, and Harish Hirani. Modular touch free hand sanitizer by separate soap and water outlet with two sensors. Copyright Application, CMERI Ref. IPMG/Copyright/2020-21/157, 2020.
11. Imtiaz Alam, Jnanendra Prasad Maji, and Harish Hirani. System hardware architecture and electronic circuit of a touch free integrated liquid soap and water dispenser for outdoor and indoor application. Copyright Application, CMERI Ref. IPMG/Copyright/2020-21/158, 2020.
12. Jyotirmoy Karmakar, Siva Ram Krishna Vadali, and Harish Hirani. Design of a portable touch free soap-cum-water dispenser. Copyright, Ref. 036CR2020, 2020.
13. https://www.slashgear.com/coronavirus-spread-study-points-to-your-shoes-13616516/Chris Burns, April 13, 2020.
14. Swarup Ranjan Debbarma, Aman Arora, Ajay Kumar Gupta, Debashis Das, and Harish Hirani. A process for external sanitizing of human body by creation of disinfectant mist over the pathway utilizing hydraulic pump. Copyright, Ref. 035CR2020, 2020.
15. Malay Kumar Karmakar, Swarup Ranjan Debbarma, Aman Arora, Chanchal Loha, and Harish Hirani. Pneumatic variant disinfection walkway unit for human body. Provisional Patent Application, CSIR Ref.0079NF2020, 2020.
16. van Doremalen, N., Bushmaker, T., Morris, Dylan H., Holbrook, Myndi G ., Gamble, A. et al. Aerosol and Surface Stability of SARS-CoV-2 as Compared with SARS-CoV-1. *The New England Journal of Medicine*, 382(16): 1564–1567, 2020, DOI: 10.1056/NEJMc2004973.
17. Lalgopal Das, Palash Kumar Maji, Bittogopal Mondal, Harish Hirani, and Sandeep Jain. Tractor mounted road sanitizing unit. Copyright, Ref. 037CR2020, 2020.
18. Dipankar Chatterjee, Samik Dutta, Bittagopal Mondal, and Harish Hirani. On the effectiveness of a "tractor mounted road sanitizing unit" designed to combat COVID-19 spread. *Journal of the Institution of Engineers (India): Series C*, 101:1093–1098, 2020, DOI 10.1007/s40032-020-00613-3.
19. Malay Kumar Karmakar, Dilpreet Singh, Sandeep Jain, Vinay Tigga, and Harish Hirani. Pneumatically operated mobile indoor disinfection unit.

Provisional Patent Application, CSIR-CMERI Ref. IPMG/Patent/2020-21/169, 2020.
20. Avinash Kumar Yadav, Dilpreet Singh, Sanjit Mukherjee, Anmol Khalko, and Harish Hirani. Battery powered disinfectant sprayer. Provisional Patent Application, CSIR-CMERI Ref. IPMG/Patent/2020-21/172, 2020
21. https://www.path.org/articles/year-covid-19-medical-oxygen-scarcity-still-costing-lives/, 2022
22. Sanjay Hasdah, Kalyan Chatterjee, and Harish Hirani. Intelligent control for mechanical ventilator. Copyright Application, CMERI Ref. IPMG/Copyright/2020-21/163, 2020.
23. Atanu Maity, Sabyasachi Mosan, Ashok Kumar Prasad, Subrata Kumar Mandal, and Harish Hirani. Hospital assistive device. Design Registration, CMERI Ref. CSIR-CMERI/IPMG/DR/2020-21/52, 2020.
24. Bittagopal Mondal, Santu Kumar Giri, Pallab Chatterjee, Siddeswar Sen, and Harish Hirani. Vehicle sanitizing unit. Copyright Application, CMERI Ref. IPMG/Copyright/2020-21/168, 2020.

Chapter 3

Water, sanitation and waste management solutions to contain the pandemic

The entire planet has been ravaged by pandemics time and again. These pandemics range from plagues of the Medieval Ages to the Spanish flu of the 20th century. To deal with pandemics effectively, there is a need to solve the contradiction "to be together" and "to be isolated". As per latest observations [1], it is mandated to isolate a patient completely from social contact and separate the items used by them. As per these studies "Covid infected persons should eat in their room, wash dishes and utensils themselves, maintain separate bedroom and bathroom". In fact, keeping "social norms" (clean and disinfect contact surfaces such as tablets, touch screens, keyboards, remote controls, keep surface wet by spreading disinfectant for a period of time, and make wearing facemasks a habit), good ventilation at home and a clean environment (minimize pollution and existence of pathogens in air) are strong local level measures required to improve the health. If possible, visits to hospitals should be minimized and intensive care health workers should implement all the measures (disinfecting shoes, mobile, clothes, hair, hot shower, etc.). These kinds of sanitization measures need to be incorporated in daily life to stop the pandemic spread rate.

Another study [2] indicates that asymptomatic individuals also can spread the pandemic. There is a very high percentage of asymptomatic infected persons (those who are a contagion but will be invisible to the system), which increases the chances of mortality of every senior citizen or person having comorbidities (pre-existing conditions of hypertension, diabetes, cardiac diseases). It can be said that the pandemic impacts all segments of the society, including all genders, young and old, migrant workers and persons with disabilities. In such situation, obvious questions related to the possibility of "in-person meeting", "group activities", "hygiene of frequently touched surfaces", "governments, private sectors, civil society and academia working together", "effective strategies for immediate deployment to broaden the scope of civic management", etc. keep coming to mind, time and again. To answer such questions, there is a need to decide an overall "social protection strategy" to fight against the pandemic by staying engaged (through S&T developments), confident and motivated.

DOI: 10.1201/9781003331179-3

As per the report [3], one of the preventive measures against pandemic is frequent hand washing. The dirt on hands may contain innumerable viruses and bacteria, and usage of soap becomes essential to remove most of the virus and bacteria completely. But as per one study [4], the novel mutated viruses can thrive in untreated waste for over a month. Thus, the water purification architecture is bound to be incorporated at local levels to tackle pandemics of such scale. In the light of the current scenario, optimum management of municipal solid and liquid wastes is the key to effectively handling the pandemic scenario and to therefore creating a pandemic resilient ecology.

3.1 INFLUENCES OF PANDEMICS ON WATER AND SANITATION SERVICES

It is unfortunate to know that many houses do not have piped waterline and residents access water through public water utilities (i.e., tube well, hand pump), fountains, etc. Many cities currently do not have access to waste collection services and they dump their untreated waste on to the city's streets and nearby streams, leading to the growing pollution of the environment. Most colonies with septic tanks have a settled sewerage system, where solid part of the waste is settled on-site in an interceptor tank while wastewater is allowed to flow out into rivers. It has been noticed that small scale vegetable farms use untreated sewage water to grow vegetables, which is more than 50% of the vegetables sold in the city. Due to shortage of water supply, the number of local farmers using untreated wastewater is growing.

Contamination of groundwater aquifers with fecal bacteria/viruses makes them unusable for household purposes [5]. As a result of this insufficient provision of hygienic services, the country may face the outbreak of waterborne diseases. Removal of virus (pathogen) from wastewater, improving the sewerage grid and appropriate treatment at the local level are essential. As these kinds of problems will vary from location to location, local community management is expected to play a major role. Integrating the whole process with the issues of sustainability and decentralization is required.

To thoroughly understand the influence of a pandemic on water, one should consider the example of COVID-19. The pandemic-infected individuals are usually quarantined/isolated in isolation wards/quarantine facilities, where strict hygiene/personal protective equipment (PPE) protocols are followed. But the wastewater discharged from the toilets/washrooms, containing traces of the virus, gets mixed with other drainage pipelines/sewers. The sanitation workers, engaged in cleaning those sewers may get in direct contact with this lethal virus. If sewer pipes are broken/cracked then there is a possibility of contamination of the underground water reserves.

As per one study [6], it has been established that wastewater and sewage water are among the potent carriers of the Novel Coronavirus. As per one more study related to some of the prominent water bodies in and around the vicinity of Hyderabad [6], it has been concluded that SARS-CoV2 was detected in all the wastewater samples collected [6]. Thus, appropriate antiviral treatment of wastewater is an indispensable aspect of the anti-pandemic strategy. The wastewater treatment facility prioritizes virus decontamination from water before it is further processed for purification based on other parameters, through effective disinfection mechanisms. A continuous and reliable monitoring program is required for the information about the water quality before its usage in various applications.

3.1.1 Science by local authorities for society

Individuals and communities have started relying too much on governments and corporations' elites to do many of the things that they once did for themselves. In other words, societies have turned to highly centralized facilities and started depending on capital-intensive sophisticated technologies to address even day-to-day common problems. This has become counterproductive, in many places, as machines require maintenance and in the absence of which machines may fail without prior warning. Additionally, those machines lack features of addressing emerging problems, like COVID-19. To achieve continuous innovations and operational improvement, the government may frame guidelines to involve society with the private sector so that a healthy, fair and sustainable developed market economy can be created. With such collective vision and allowing society to play a part of management, a self-sufficient fair community can prevail.

It appears that COVID-19 is serving as a golden opportunity for people to re-engage as society and care for each other instead of staying alone and independent. It is worth mentioning that people can create local solutions to their problems by changing their behavior in response to today's economic and social conditions. By doing so, they can form more democratic, self-reliant societies. If society is encouraged to take pride in self-sufficiency and nurture knowledgebase, then finding jobs within local communities will not be difficult.

Technological institutions, public-funded R&D laboratories and universities have been researching so that the efforts of their S&T practitioners can positively influence society during unforeseen global crises. There is a need to spread scientific knowledgebase among society stakeholders and establish a collaborative science by local authorities for society (SLS) model for better provision of sanitation services and accountability.

3.2 MECHANIZED DRAINAGE CLEANING AND ON-SITE WASTEWATER PURIFICATION TECHNOLOGIES

With an ever increasing population, the supply of water has become much less than its demand. With the increase in water scarcity, food supply and industrial growth will be hampered. Therefore, efforts have been made to harvest water in many ways to meet the demand. For example, farmers in towns/cities often use untreated wastewater to grow vegetables and fruits. The wastewater comprises water rejected from households and industries. Household wastewater may contain biodegradable materials, nitrogen, phosphorus, potassium, dissolved minerals, toxic chemicals and pathogens. The presence of stable organics, namely, phenols, pesticides, chlorinated hydrocarbons may cause many serious problems creating a toxic environment. The dissolved inorganic substances in the form of total dissolved solid (TDS) and compounds based on Na, Ca, Mg, etc. may also cause salinity and associated adverse effects in soil. The presence of heavy metals beyond their permissible limit is a highly worrying factor as they are not only identified as toxic for plants and animals but also create many adverse health issues for humans. Very importantly, the presence of pathogens, like viruses, bacteria, helminth eggs, fecal coliforms, etc. must be taken care of as they may cause many communal diseases. Thereby, the use of wastewater without proper treatment would be highly undesirable and unhealthy [7]. There are a number of ways, which can be opted for testing (chemical analysis and some pathogenic bacteria tests) and water treatment to make urban wastewater suitable for irrigation purposes. The reduction in leakage and avoidance of untreated wastewater for irrigation can be achieved by localizing the water purification services.

The impact of contaminants present in wastewater for agricultural use must be investigated before the utilization [8]. The excess nitrogen content in water delays the agricultural growing season and its maturity, thereby causing economic loss to farmers. Furthermore, excessive amounts of N and P increase growth of undesirable aquatic species known as eutrophication.

In most of the developing countries, which are more vulnerable to the impact of a pandemic, cleaning of drainage/sewage systems through manual scavenging, that too once in a while, is a conventional practice which violates the principles of human dignity and hygiene standards. To help society, there is a need for technological innovation in the form of a mechanized mobile drainage cleaning system, which collects water and passes it through a sieve membrane filtration system to separate the bigger particles. The mechanization of the sanitation infrastructure is required to avoid the chances of contamination, which occur due to manual handling and direct contact. Two different sketches of the mechanized drainage cleaning system-cum-wastewater treatment plant are shown in Figure 3.1. The salient features of such systems are:

- Vehicle-mounted modular mechanized sewage cleaning system.
- Extraction of slurry from the manhole opening.
- Floating material separation system from sewerage water.
- Cleaning system of sewerage water for reuse in a pressure jet.
- High pressure water jet-based blockage clearing system.

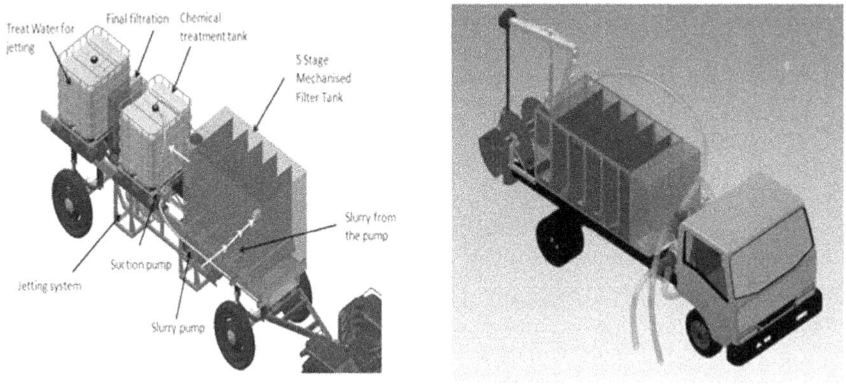

Tractor attached drain cleaning system

Truck chassis mounted drain cleaning system

Figure 3.1 Schematic diagram of the drainage cleaning system.

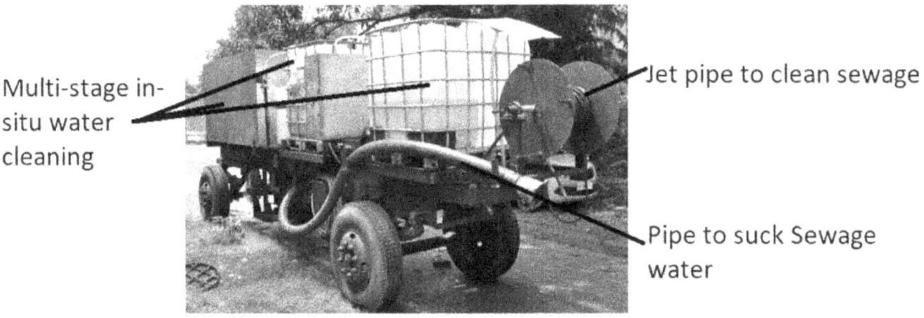

Figure 3.2 Developed mechanized drainage cleaning system.

Figure 3.2 shows a mechanized drainage cleaning system and the process flow of the system given in Figure 3.3. Regular cleaning of manholes and drains will reduce the effective water requirements. In addition, there is a need to reuse the wastewater. Various methodologies have been used since the 20th century for municipal wastewater treatment to control water contaminations (e.g., harmful heavy metals, total coliform, fecal coliform) and provide sustainable solutions for the usage in community for household and agricultural purposes. The reuse of industrial wastewater, in which the effluents are discharged by industry plants, is out of the scope of this book. The present subheading describes use of municipal wastewater, which is a combination of sewer or sanitary sewer generated by domestic uses of water and contains feces or urine from people's toilets, several pathogens, bacteria, metals, etc. In other words, the municipal water consists mostly of gray water (water from sinks, bathtubs, bathrooms, showers, washing machines),

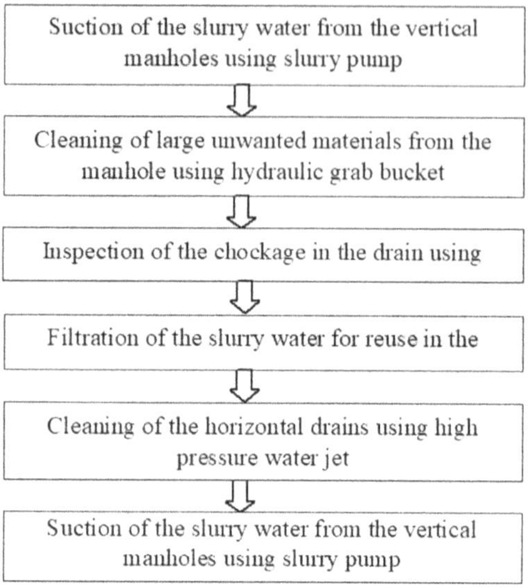

Suction of the slurry water from the vertical manholes using slurry pump
Cleaning of large unwanted materials from the manhole using hydraulic grab bucket
Inspection of the chockage in the drain using
Filtration of the slurry water for reuse in the
Cleaning of the horizontal drains using high pressure water jet
Suction of the slurry water from the vertical manholes using slurry pump

Figure 3.3 Process flow of the mechanized drainage cleaning system.

Physical Treatment	Chemical Treatment	Biological Treatment
• Sedimentation • Aeration • Froth Flotation • Screening	• Adsorption • Chlorine dosing • Coagulation • Ozonation • Neutralization	• UV treatment • Oxidation

Figure 3.4 Wastewater treatment methodologies.

black water (water combined with human waste, which is flushed away), soaps and detergents and toilet paper.

The reuse of municipal wastewater after proper treatment for agriculture or domestic use is highly necessary to meet the demand of growing population [9, 10] and reduce the demand for freshwater resources. The basic methodologies (Figure 3.4) for the wastewater treatment process can be categorized into three processes: physical, chemical and biological [11].

The physical processes, as depicted in Figure 3.1, involve the removal of solid particles/debris by sedimentation or screening through different meshes of diverse pore sizes. The chemical processes mostly involve chlorination and reacting with dissolved/undissolved inorganic/organic contaminants. The physical and chemical processes can be sequentially combined as shown in Figure 3.1. For example, by adding alum into wastewater, certain anionic pollutants coagulate together into large heavier masses and can be removed faster through physical processes. In addition, certain dissolved organic chemicals can be effectively separated out by adsorbing in activated carbon-based filters. The removal of bacteria, viruses and other microorganisms in water can be very effectively done by proper UV treatment and ozone treatment processes.

Farmers are often happy to use the partially treated wastewater as it contains nitrogen and phosphorus elements, which may increase the yield of agricultural plants compared to plants irrigated with fresh water. However, the risk to plants due to the presence of some pathogens causing diseases (e.g., diarrhea, dysentery, typhoid, and cholera) must be considered. Therefore, there is a need to account for the reverse effect of treated wastewater particularly its usage in the irrigation of edible crops [12]. To prevent transmission of pathogens, efficient microbiological quality guidelines and appropriate standards for reuse of treated wastewater in agriculture must be established. Zero levels of fecal coli bacteria and fecal streptococci in treated wastewater are a preferable choice [13]. To achieve these kinds of standards, multi-stage purification is required. Mechanical filtration is used as a primary treatment procedure and chemical treatment is performed subsequently. More details on water treatment are provided in Annexure-II.

To summarize, a wastewater plant can be developed with a multistep filtration procedure as per the standard methods, including mechanical screening, aeration, chlorination, activated carbon filtration and finally UV treatment to filter off any solid or dissolved materials in the form of organic as well as inorganic compounds and kill microorganisms including bacteria, viruses and other pathogens and treat wastewater properly without any compromise. Decentralized sewerage management systems and water purification can provide employment opportunities, as these kinds of services at the local level provide even more benefits compared to centralized sewerage management systems. Governments can incentivize by providing partial support to the start-ups and may allow the companies to generate money for these kinds of services by charging a nominal amount to the public. The policy of charging some nominal price on "modernized" sanitation services will be useful for overall social growth and provide an image of modernity and progress. The idea is that if the private sector is given enough motivation in upgrading waste processing technologies, the sector itself would come up with the best way to solve local problems and upgrade current hygiene standards to a level, whereby contamination and transmission can be arrested to a major extent, even in the post-pandemic era.

3.3 MUNICIPAL SOLID WASTE AND ITS RELATION WITH PANDEMIC

Municipal solid waste (MSW) consists of everyday items that have value for the public before their use and after their usage get discarded such as food waste, horticulture waste, plastics, paper, rags, bottles, electronic waste, inert waste consisting of construction and demolition debris and so on. Horticulture waste includes street sweepings, tree trimmings, wastes from parks, beaches and other recreational areas. The major sources for this type of waste are households, schools, colleges, businesses and municipal services. Household and commercial solid waste consists of food waste, tires, paper, cardboard, rags, glass, metals, polymer waste such as plastic and inert waste such as ash, consumer electronics, batteries, etc. Institutional solid waste includes plastic, paper, cardboard, food waste, glass, metals wastes. Therefore, the major types of MSW are food waste, paper, plastic, rags, metal and glass, electric light bulbs, batteries, discarded medicines and automotive parts [14].

The MSW is a menace all throughout the globe. One obvious question comes to mind: does infrastructure to manage the waste such as collection, segregation, storage, transportation, processing and disposal exist? Sometimes municipalities simply dump the waste and claim these dumps are landfills. In a few days' to a few months' time, smoke rises steadily from the landfill piles, as the decomposing waste generates highly combustible methane gas. Sometimes fire breaks out at landfills, which severely compromises air quality in the city. Due to lack of jobs, people get involved in picking sorted waste from landfill areas that too without any protective gloves and often cut themselves on bits of glass and remain vulnerable to infections and illnesses. This is a clear indication of a flawed system of waste disposal and management. Ideally, there should not be any landfill area and waste must be processed within a few hours of its creation. Such decentralized waste management, where segregated waste gets treated locally that too in a few hours of time, is the requirement.

The traditional methods of waste collection and dumping in trucks/tractors accelerate the spread of the pandemic. The sanitation workers and the rag pickers associated directly with handling of solid waste are most susceptible to a variety of infectious and chronic diseases. The situation is even worse due to the COVID-19 pandemic as used facemasks, gloves, etc. from households are being dumped with the regular household garbage. Unscientific management of this waste can lead to deterioration of the situation further and unforeseen adverse effects of new pandemic on human health and the environment may emerge. The safe handling, management and final disposal of these wastes are therefore a vital element in an effective "social protection strategy".

During the pandemic at the beginning a lockdown was imposed as a preventive measure to combat the spread of virus. However, despite the lockdown, there was always a steady rise in the number of new cases and deaths every day. Although containment zones were identified to restrict the spread of the virus, appropriate measure to prevent dissemination of the virus through the municipal waste was lacking. The key to efficient and healthy waste management in this public health emergency situation of pandemic lies in the mechanized segregation of waste into different components in a decentralized manner ensuring minimal human intervention. ZERO waste residential complexes can be achieved through appropriate technologies for safe disposal and conversion into value-added products. Treatment of solid waste in localized premises will break the chain of pandemic from spreading across the cities.

To overcome the challenges faced with the current solid waste management system, integrated municipal solid waste plants can be designed and developed. In the plant, daily waste generated from the residential campus can be collected with appropriate measures and processed in an environment-friendly way to achieve a ZERO waste campus. The main element of such a plant is the mechanized segregation of municipal solid waste, in which the contactless segregation operation is carried out. The triple treatment therapy consists of spraying a solution of sodium hypochlorite in the waste following UV-C treatment prior to mechanized segregation following preheating of waste using hot air at 60°C utilizing a recuperative air preheater to inactivate microorganisms contained in the waste including coronavirus. The separated garbage such as biodegradable waste including garden waste, non-biodegradable polymer waste including plastic, facemasks, gloves, etc. is treated and disposed off at the pilot plant, thereby disrupting the outward movement of solid waste and breaking of the chain to prevent the spread of virus through solid waste management routes. The overall system is easy to operate and maintain with bare minimum manpower involvement and is self-sustainable in terms of operational energy requirement. The salient features of such system include:

1. Decentralized solid waste management plant: Disposal of solid waste in localized premises toward breaking the chain of virus and combat its spread.
2. Disinfection of solid waste with sodium hypochlorite and UV-C treatment.
3. Mechanized segregation of solid waste: No manual handling.
4. Thermal treatment of solid waste during the segregation process.
5. Collection of segregated products through the UV-C gateway.
6. Disposal of polymer waste (including facemasks, gloves, etc.) through the pyrolysis process.
7. Disposal of organic waste through biogasification and pellets.
8. Self-sustainable systems in terms of operational energy.
9. Minimum manpower involvement and easy to maintain.

3.3.1 Centralized–decentralized model dichotomy

A centralized management system refers to a "centralized approach" in which an individual or a small group of people participate in planning, decision-making, implementation, monitoring and evaluation of any initiative/intervention whereas a "decentralized management system" pertains to involvement of all primary stakeholders (community) in the decision-making, implementation, monitoring and evaluation of the program/initiative/activity. With growing volume of municipal garbage, decentralized community level waste management systems are preferred to reduce the burden of handling large volumes of MSW at a centralized location. Some of the advantages of decentralized waste management are:

- Decentralized systems require lower levels of mechanization than the centralized solutions and provide manufacturing opportunities to small entrepreneurs (the manufacturing sector becomes a generator of direct jobs instead of a wealth generator).
- Decentralized options can be optimized (in terms of efficiency/utility) for the local waste type.
- Collection and transportation costs in decentralized systems are reduced substantially.

Figures 3.5 and 3.6 represent drawbacks of centralized waste processing and advantages of the decentralized waste processing, respectively.

3.3.2 Innovative segregation of waste through a mechanized model

Municipal solid waste is classified into two categories (a) live waste and (b) dead waste. The wastes which are being collected daily by the municipalities are termed as "live waste". The wastes which have been dumped over the landfill site are termed as "dead waste".

The mechanized segregation system can be developed for segregation of both live and dead wastes into different segments. The segregation process starts with dumping of solid waste material into a bin directly from the dumper carrying the materials. The segregation system is capable of segregating metallic waste (metal body, metal container, etc.), biodegradable waste (foods, vegetables, fruits, grass, etc.), non-biodegradable (plastics, packaging material, pouches, bottles, etc.) and inert (glass, stones, etc.) wastes. Figure 3.7 shows the process layout of the segregation system for live waste.

The municipal solid waste contains a high amount of moisture. The high moisture content will reduce the efficiency of mechanized sorting. In the presence of moisture, the biodegradation rate increases causing release of CO_2 and methane, so it is necessary to reduce the garbage moisture in a

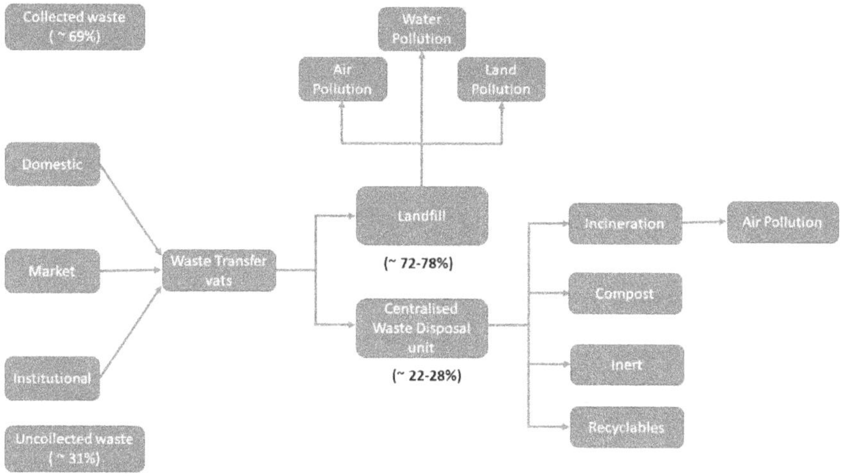

Figure 3.5 Drawbacks of conventional centralized waste processing.

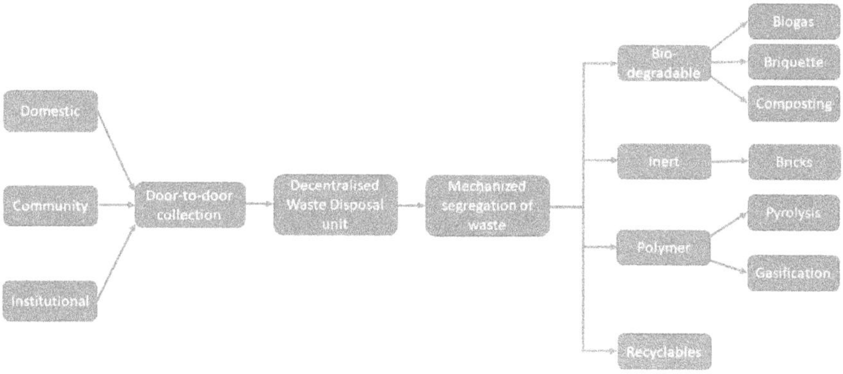

Figure 3.6 Advantages of decentralized waste processing.

short span of time. Therefore, MSW is passed over a horizontal roller conveyor where it is exposed to hot air (60–75°C) to reduce moisture contents. The dried material is passed over a rotary magnetic drum separator where the iron components (Fe) separate out which are collected in a hopper for reuse. The rest of the materials are passed over an eddy current separator where non-ferrous metallic parts (Al, Cu) are separated out. The remaining wastes are sent to the air separation unit where the lighter particles (plastics, paper) and heavy mass (biomass) are being separated. The lighter objects (plastics, paper) are directly fed into a shredder. The shredded material will be sent to the polymer waste pyrolysis unit using a vibratory chute for pyrolysis operation. The segregated biomass can be utilized for production

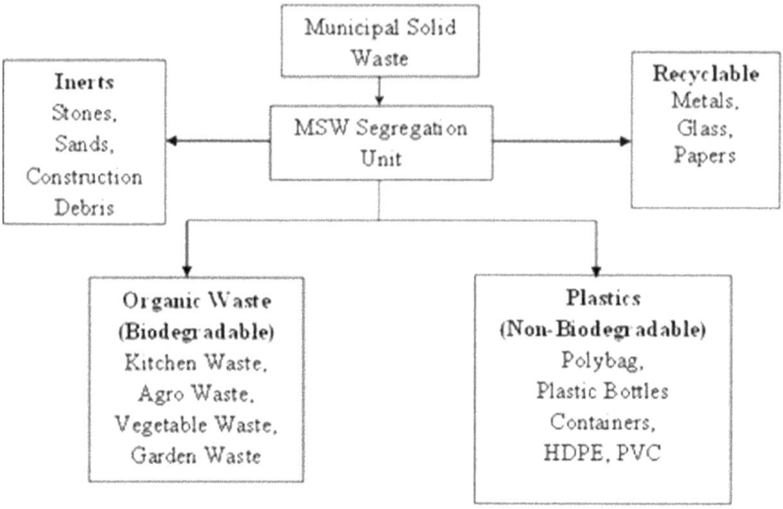

Figure 3.7 The process layout of the segregation system for live waste.

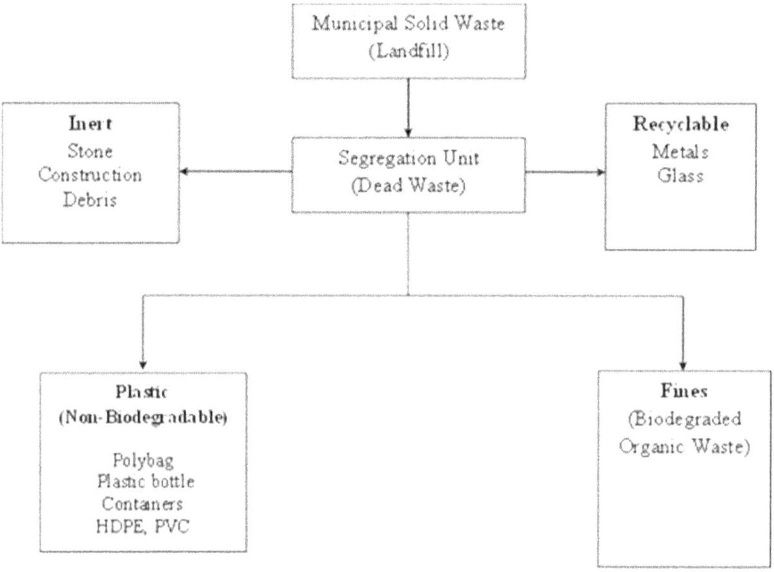

Figure 3.8 The process layout of the segregation system for dead waste.

of biogas in the biomethanation unit through a grinder. Mechanized segregation units of capacities 50 kg/h and 100 kg/h are shown in Annexure-II. The process flow of the mechanized segregation unit for dead waste developed is shown in Figure 3.8.

3.3.3 Salient novelties of the biogas, sludge and composting processes

Biogas production from animal excreta such as cow dung is a well-developed technology. Different technological interventions can be incorporated to make the biogas production process from segregated organic waste more mechanized and efficient. A biomass grinder-cum-stirrer can be developed as a single unit where grinding (requires high speed) and stirring (requires slow speed) can be done simultaneously. An automatic gas evacuation system senses the position of the floating dome, eliminating the manual intervention for gas collection in a storage tank. Recycling of the slurry water improves the gas production yield and reduces fresh water consumption. The combustion efficiency of slurry from organic waste is generally higher and it can be used as combustion as well as binding material for preparation of biomass briquettes.

The technology can be developed for production of concentrated biomass briquettes with higher bulk density and volumetric energy density utilizing shredded leaves, dust from dead twigs and other forms of waste such as charcoal fines in a simple single extrusion die screw press. The ratio of different components like shredded leaves, dust from dead twigs, charcoal fines and slurry in the mixture forming the briquette is obtained resulting is better combustion properties like slow burning and a higher heating value and improved emission characteristics in regards to formation of smoke, soot and other noxious gases such as carbon monoxide and oxides of nitrogen. The emission characteristics of such briquettes are also within limit. These technologies, if implemented in a decentralized manner, can reduce the requirement of liquified petroleum gas (LPG). The slurry, obtained from anaerobic degradation of wet waste, can also be used primarily as manure or fertilizer in field and can be used as a binder material for briquettes.

3.3.4 Disposal of plastic waste through pyrolysis

As plastic is non-biodegradable, inappropriately disposed plastics get dumped in oceans. To avoid it, the pyrolysis process, which is a waste to energy technology converting waste plastics under anaerobic conditions into gas, oil, and char products, may be explored. Technology for obtaining diesel equivalent fuel from crude oil can also be developed locally. Figure 3.9 represents the schematic process layout for plastic pyrolysis. More details of plastic pyrolysis are provided in Annexure-II.

3.3.5 Disposal of plastic waste utilizing high temperature plasma

Plasma arc technology is eco-friendly but is a less explored technology for proper disposal of the mountain of solid waste material generated on a

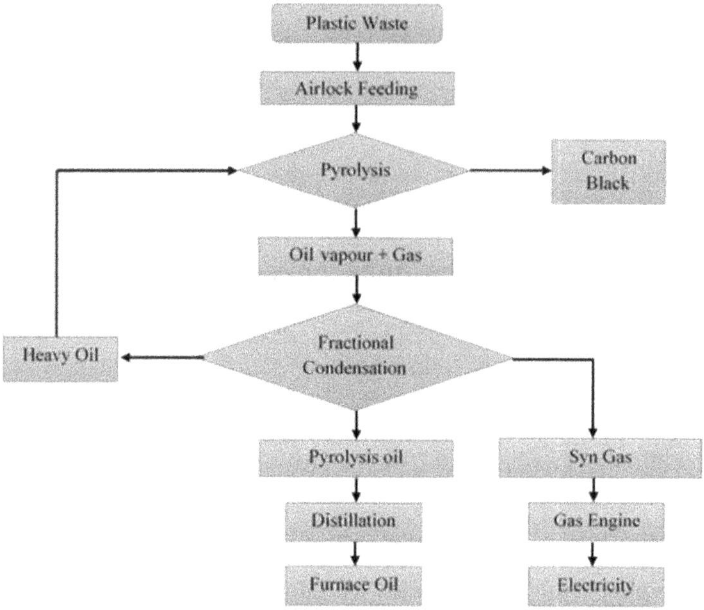

Figure 3.9 The schematic process layout for plastic pyrolysis into a gas engine.

daily basis. In this technology, electrical ionization between two electrodes cathode and anode at low voltage (30–50 V) and high current (300–400 A) is being used to treat the waste at a temperature as high as ~3000°C using a plasma torch. At such a high temperature, the generated output gases are mainly CO, H_2, hydrocarbons and CO_2. The chances of generation of carcinogenic gases at such elevated temperatures are remote. The CO and H_2 enriched syngas has a high calorific value. The product gas after passing through the plasma treatment is made to pass through the carbon sieves (REDOX reactor). This will help to convert carbon from the sieve and oxygen (may be entrapped from linkages and breaking of water vapor) to form CO and CO_2. A catalytic converter shall be used to convert any traces of hydrocarbon into CO and H_2. Catalysts like nickel can be used for this purpose. The gas is then cleaned in a cyclone separator and scrubber and subsequently cooled in a condenser. This CO and H_2 enriched syngas has a high calorific value. This gas will be primarily stored into a gas holder and will be used for generation of electricity after combustion into a gas engine. The process layout is shown in Figure 3.10 and the plastic disposal unit of 25 kg/h capacity developed is shown in Figure 3.11.

This less explored technology is proficient compared to other conventional techniques like landfilling and incineration, etc. Incineration can cause potential emission of toxic pollutants like dioxin, furan, SO_x and NO_x among others. Incineration cannot be used for all kinds of wastes

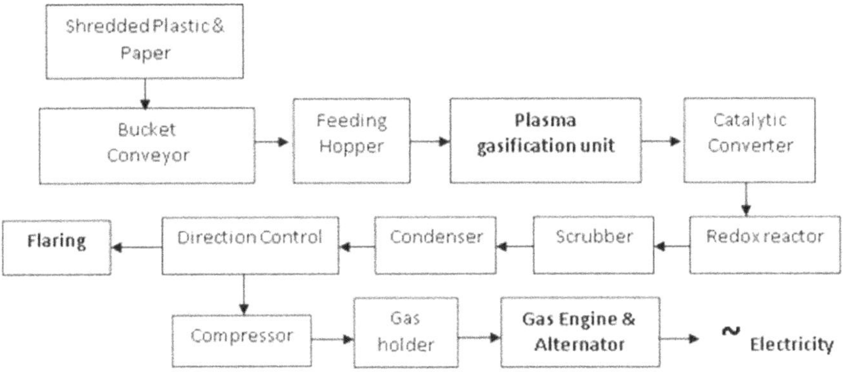

Figure 3.10 The process layout of the plasma gasification unit.

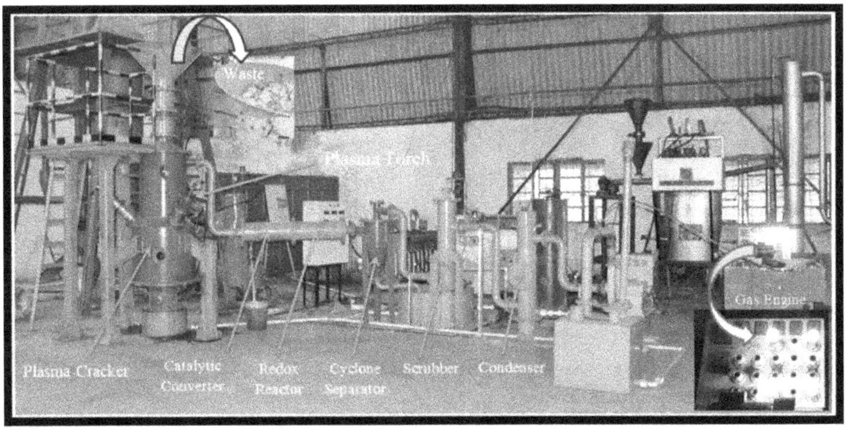

Figure 3.11 The plastic disposal unit (capacity: 25 kg/h).

and it needs waste with high calorific values for combustion. In addition, incineration requires moisture content in waste to be less than 50% and a sufficient amount of oxygen to fully oxidize the fuel. Similarly, landfilling can cause air as well as water pollution through leaching of contaminants into ground as well as surface water. The plasma-assisted arc-driven technology is superior to most of the waste management technologies practiced in modern day to date.

More details of integrated waste management are provided in Annexure-II. Effective decentralized waste management may reduce pollution and contribute toward achieving a safe and healthy environment. Government ought to encourage companies to deploy decentralized waste management facilities in various locations and boost green economy. The advances in science and technology need to be harnessed to create a robust environment for living. In a cleaner environment, medical expenditure may reduce drastically and productivity of work may increase.

3.3.6 Scientific and technological advancements

- Biomass resources such as leaves and wood are abundantly available in most of the developing countries. It constitutes the major source of energy in rural households for cooking and heating purposes. Burning of loose biomass leads to an increase in the level of indoor air pollutants such as particulate matters, soot particles and noxious gases such as carbon monoxide. The adverse effect of biomass as cooking fuel is primarily due to poor handling properties of the loose biomass, i.e., low volumetric energy density due to low bulk density and associated inhomogeneous structure. Therefore, the developed technology for production of concentrated biomass briquettes with higher bulk density and volumetric energy density utilizing shredded leaves, dust from dead twigs and other forms of waste such as charcoal fines in a simple single extrusion die screw press will be very useful.
- Development and selection of components for mechanized segregation of municipal solid waste through mass and energy balance diagrams considering physical composition of waste. Selection of different process parameters, like conveyor speed, amount of moisture to be removed from the solid waste, speed of blowers, are selected through rigorous experimentation.
- Development of a plasma torch to maintain the temperature inside the plasma cracker around 3000°C and maintaining an oxygen-starved environment inside the cracker to prevent the formation of any toxic gases.
- Development of technology for production of biomethane from segregated organic waste: Different technological interventions have been incorporated to make the biogas production process more mechanized and efficient.
- Effective handling of landfill or dead waste and possibilities for clearing landfills.
- Generation of biogas from the segregated organic waste and utilization of the same for household and commercial purposes as an alternative to LPG/compressed natural gas (CNG) reduces import burden.
- Eco-friendly disposal of sanitary waste through high temperature plasma-assisted arc-driven technology with minimal level toxin emission.

BIBLIOGRAPHY

1. https://www.cdc.gov/coronavirus/2019-ncov/if-you-are-sick/isolation.html, 2022
2. https://www.healthline.com/health-news/people-without-symptoms-carry-just-as-much-covid-19-as-symptomatic-people, 2022
3. https://www.mohfw.gov.in/pdf/GuidelinesforHomeIsolationofverymildpresymptomaticCOVID19cases.pdf, 2022
4. Poulomi Roy. *Waste Water Treatment: An Unavoidable Solution to COVID-19.* CSIR-CMERI, Durgapur, 2021.
5. S.R. Crane, and J.A. Moore. Bacterial pollution of groundwater: a review. *Water, Air, & Soil Pollution*, 22:67–83, 1984.
6. https://www.ccmb.res.in/presscovrg/Waste_water_COVID-19_surveillance.pdf, 2022
7. S. Al-Salem Saqer. Environmental considerations for wastewater reuse in agriculture. *Water Science and Technology*, 33(10–11):345–353, 1996.
8. R Andricevic, and V. Cvetkovic. Evaluation of risk from contaminants migrating by groundwater. *Water Resources Research*, 32(3):611–621, 1996.
9. Mohamed F. Hamoda, and Saed M. Al-Awadi. Improvement of effluent quality for reuse in a dairy farm. *Water Science and Technology*, 33(10–11):79–85, 1996.
10. B. Heinzmann, and F. Sarfert. An integrated water management concept to ensure a safe water supply and high drinking water quality on an ecologically sound basis. *Water Science and Technology*, 31(8):281–291, 1995.
11. Office of Wastewater Management Washington DC. *Primer for Municipal Wastewater Treatment Systems.* EPA 832-R-04-001, 2004.
12. S. Toze. Reuse of effluent water – benefits and risks. *Agricultural Water Management*, 80(2005):147–159, 2005.
13. Khaled S. Balkhair. Microbial contamination of vegetable crop and soil profile in arid regions under controlled application of domestic wastewater. *Saudi Journal of Biological Sciences*, 23(1):S83–S92, 2016.
14. Evaluation and Oversight Unit, UNEP. *UNEP Annual Evaluation Report*, 2004.

Chapter 4

Farm mechanization as a recovery path toward sustainable growth

Every pandemic situation brings not only a period of global health issues, but a time span of significant economic crisis also. The main emphasis should be on containing and mitigating the pandemic disease itself, but the economic impacts are also considerable. The supply chain mechanisms are severely affected. Thousands of small suppliers who supply mid-sized suppliers go through stages of collapsing. Such a recession rapidly increases unemployment and social inequality. Fragmented societies, less revenue and higher lending volume pose existential threat to government organizations. Though the government takes several measures to safeguard the economy, only few companies find their way toward understanding, reacting to and learning lessons from rapidly unfolding pandemic events and reintegrate their functioning, but many micro, small and medium enterprises (MSMEs) being financially fragile find it difficult to survive. Hiring full-time employees costs significantly more than equivalent independent part time staff and this makes companies keep a low headcount of full-time employees. Perhaps there is a need to reinvent business strategies to reduce social inequality and create ample jobs for self-sustainability. It is important to note that agriculture, manufacturing and associated services are the biggest job-creating sectors. In the present chapter, farm mechanization has been deliberated. In the next chapter, manufacturing and associated services are described.

To boost the economic prospects of the concerned, government aligns the financial institutions to extend the best possible financial support to the start-ups and the MSMEs. Many unemployed youths would like to start their own micro, small or medium business depending on their knowledgebase and financial support. Those young entrepreneurs have a lot of potential and can do well for the economic growth of the country; but most of their business ideas fail and are unable to attract funding agencies. There is a need to initiate the spread of science and technology across those entrepreneurs so that they learn the mistakes by technical analysis and make good products/processes by rectifying those mistakes. Theoretical technical knowledge is not sufficient enough; practical skills and high-level proficiency are also required.

DOI: 10.1201/9781003331179-4

It has become necessary for the R&D laboratories to prioritize the interests of start-ups and MSMEs while launching new products/services related directly or indirectly for the larger benefit of the society. The public R&D laboratories may assist in poverty alleviation through development of new technologies that increase opportunities for increasing incomes of MSMEs. The technology pricing profile must also get aligned to the needs of the micro and small enterprises (MSEs) and rural small businesses. The procedure to nurture the new/micro industries must be specified. In addition, the start-ups and MSEs are urged to come forward and join hands with R&D institutions to enhance the economic and societal profile of their enterprises.

Government can subsidize many business sectors (i.e., agriculture, localized hygiene and sanitation services, medical assistive devices, water purification services, municipal waste management services, etc.), which are vital to the economy and for the well-being of the nation. The agriculture sector is one of the most vital sectors for the government and it can provide all support to farm industries contributing to food security and provide subsidies on environmentally friendly food processing technologies. Farmers or young entrepreneurs working in the farm sector must understand that farming is a business. With the growing framework to provide IT-based services, it is recommended to provide services to farmers. The services may include early warning systems for rain, advisory on the harvest time, pest control, enhancing crop yields, etc.

A major constraint during pandemic is disruptions in the supply chain of the necessary items/components. Digital internet-based services by prospective suppliers/traders/business units provide time-bound services to empower stakeholders and help the society at large. All manufacturing industries can adopt digital logistics platforms for integrating marketing, payment and fast-track physical delivery from the warehouse to the customer. But delivery staffs interact with a number of customers and create a vector for spreading the virus. To reduce these risks, the developed COVID protection system (COPS) (described in Chapter 2, subheading 2.8), equipped with a facemask delivery system, touchless handwash, disinfectants, temperature checks, vehicle wash, must be installed at community gates of all the societies to break the virus chain. Government can provide funds for R&D, deployment and nurturing business units in the form of partial grants and loans at favorable interest rates and its consequent liabilities can be indemnified by government.

4.1 FORMING PARTNERSHIPS WITH COMMUNITY-BASED ORGANIZATIONS

It is necessary to collectively mobilize resources of organizations and partner up to provide solutions to the evolving demands/requirements of the societies. In every country, there are a number of non-governmental organizations (NGOs) and self-help groups, who can play a major role in the development of social and economic aspects of the nation. Fundamental to the very character of every NGO is that it is not-for-profit, non-governmental, organized, independent, autonomous and voluntary. NGOs facilitate communication upward from individuals (i.e., what native individuals are thinking, doing and feeling) to the government and downward from the government to native folks (i.e., what the government is coming up with and doing). In some cases, NGOs become representatives of poor people and influence government policies and programs toward more social welfare. There are more than 1.5 million NGOs in the USA, 0.3 million NGOs in Brazil, 0.2 million NGOs in South Africa and more than 1.0 million NGOs in India. Emergence of civil society groups, demand for analysis-based action, trends toward increased decentralization, poor performance of few policymakers, scandals involving public officials, etc. led to the growth of NGOs.

The NGOs can bring together civil society, public-funded R&D institutions and private sectors and strengthen the country to fight against untoward economic prospects. These organizations pursue a public interest agenda such as creating employment opportunities for groups of women, the differently abled and unemployed youth aiming for the goals of poverty eradication. These organizations, operating on local, grassroots level, can be engaged to provide a forum to develop tailor-made solutions for local society to support health, safety and wellness of people. Programs that help to shape "new ways of manufacturing" and "design for environment" can be started. These initiatives can help in fortifying national manufacturing capabilities and support the clarion call of "Vocal for Local".

The NGOs can participate in manufacturing of touchless soap and water dispensing systems used for washing of hands to ensure comprehensive sanitization requisites of any organization with a considerable amount of footfall and arrest the contamination and spread of the virus/bacteria. Similarly, other products (high efficiency hydrophobic facemask, soap, sanitizer, disinfection walkway, disinfectant sprayer, mechanical ventilator with oxygen enrichment, hospital waste management facility, hospital care assistive robotic devices, COVID protection system for gated community), described in Chapter 2 of this book, can be manufactured at the local level. Start-ups with initiatives of NGOs, on a variety of products/services and available manufacturing information, can take better decisions and economy may spring back to its feet. Private companies, with the partnership of community-based organizations, can sail through uncertain times with a consolidated socioeconomic strength.

Often gross domestic product (GDP) is considered as an indicator of national growth, which is incomplete as it does not involve considerations of improving human value, conserving natural resources, minimizing inequality in the society and enhancing the well-being of the society. There is a need to focus on "sustainable developmental goals" which is a far better indicator than GDP. In this respect "sustainable agriculture" must focus on people at the bottom of the pyramid which also incorporates the social, economic and environmental aspects. Priority shall be given to renewable energy, biomass (food agriculture, forestry) and fisheries sectors. Promotion of agriculture as a high-potential and economically attractive sector via farm mechanization would be part of the solution to the youth unemployment crisis and it would also increase the overall productivity and attract private investment. The easy availability of farm machinery to the farmers/youths by establishing custom hiring centers of agricultural machinery operated by self-help groups, cooperative societies and private/rural entrepreneurs [1] will in turn increase the number of jobs. The custom hiring centers can be equipped with a series of implements that can perform all the farming operations from seedbed preparation to post-harvesting of the crops. In other words, by popularizing rental markets (i.e., farm machinery Rs. 200 per hour, operator Rs. 100 per hour), the services of tractors, power tillers, power weeders, hand-held machines, multicrop reapers, various implements and pump sets become divisible and extendable to small and marginal farm holdings. With such a development, growing two or three crops per year from the same field as farm power with appropriate timeliness is possible. As a result, the farm machines can be operated on a custom hire basis for 20–22 hours a day in three shifts. Availability of such centers will enhance the machinery usages in agriculture throughout the crop cycle which will enhance crop productivity, increase earning and decrease poverty. In addition, availability of cold storage in the rural areas helps to get better prices of vegetables and fruits. The subsidy on cold storages might help farmers overcome the lower market prices during harvest season.

There is a need to understand long-term benefit or sustainable growth. Few innovations may benefit society for short durations (few years) but impact negatively in the long run. For example, innovation of extracting ground water helped farmers in the short term, but unavailability of technologies to replenish extracted water have negative consequences for the society as a whole.

4.2 SUSTAINABILITY AND LOCAL COLLECTIVE ACTION: A FRAMEWORK

A framework can be developed with the intention to analyze the potential of communities to manage themselves for their own sustainability, meeting all the present needs while maintaining the capability to fulfill the needs of future generations. This requires focus on the environmental, social and economic balance. To develop the framework, a vision of aligning the motivation of individuals, public-funded organizations and government agencies are required. We need to establish mechanisms and implementation strategies that could galvanize them with the aim of successful transformation to a sustainable future.

Since the outbreak of COVID-19 there has been a substantial reduction in jobs and many people have lost their livelihoods. The jobless workers require a basic income to survive and exist with their dependent family members. The easiest remedy is farming, as they can get engaged in farming and produce food for themselves. In such a situation, the agriculture sector has to see a growth, minimizing the unemployment rates and forming a new agricultural force, who will ultimately lend a helping hand in shaping the country into becoming an agricultural powerhouse. But history indicates that farmers are often poor and unable to arrange food for themselves. Therefore, one needs to look at the way food is produced, processed, distributed and consumed, and innovate to lift farmers out of poverty, tackle unemployment for youth and rural women, and achieve food security. With young agricultural entrepreneurs' innovation, technology deployment, information and communication technology (ICT) skills and the range of products and services provided, there are hopes. Furthermore, as the younger generation loves automation and technology, the automated and digital farming would attract them to the agricultural field. Time has come to minimize the wastage of food by developing and deploying a number of post-harvest technological solutions. The optimum use of such technologies has the potential to bring automation in agriculture. The need of the hour is to provide support to such smaller businesses and marginalized farmers by catalyzing the agricultural momentum through low-cost mechanization in the farming processes implementing cost-effective technology innovations. The farm mechanization revolution will provide a further thrust to Industry 4.0 through an amalgamation of artificial intelligence and Internet of things.

Going beyond farm mechanization, innovations in agricultural processes, ranging from farm products to selling in markets, scaling up innovation to reach the masses, handling climate change and effective transportation, are required. All this can be achieved by including information and communication methods (ICT innovations) in the entire value chain, which in turn can create jobs for young people. In addition, employment opportunities for rural youth can be generated by supporting knowledge sharing and skill development related to horticulture and post-harvest management. These kinds of initiatives do not only create jobs, but they address social needs also including protection of the environment and natural resources and increase future productivity of the economy. The overall framework should be such that no one is left behind, especially people who are ready to work. The framework requires:

- Development, transfer, dissemination and diffusion of technology and innovation.
- Shift from "agriculture alone" to a network-based system approach that better responds to the needs of small farm holders.

- Practicing e-agriculture using information and communication technology (ICT) to exchange information, ideas and resources to improve decision-making.
- Innovative technologies and approaches to all segments of rural community to increase productivity and profitability.
- Knowledge sharing of low-cost agricultural equipment and scientific practices to promote incremental innovation on the existing technology.
- Working with small-scale enterprises, NGOs and local organizations to ensure small farmers have access to mechanized services.

4.3 FARM MECHANIZATION

Agriculture, a profession of both hope and despair, is pivotal to the world's economy and survival. A rough estimate shows that cultivation of one hectare of farmland manually (one person) requires more than one month time compared to one day time required by a mechanized seeder. This example indicates that mechanization, which covers all levels of farming and processing technologies, from simple and basic hand tools to more sophisticated and motorized equipment [2], can ease and reduce hard labor and relieve labor shortages. With the required push from the advancement in technologies and the incentives and schemes provided by the government, agriculture has started to move toward mechanization, albeit at a slow rate due to apprehensiveness of farmers to resort to new techniques and technologies and their ability to afford them. It is necessary to consider mechanization of smaller-sized equipment and involve more and more micro and small enterprises as a fabricator/manufacturer. In the following paragraphs some of technological solutions in the domain of farm machinery, having potential to support micro and small industries, are described.

4.3.1 Small tractor

A small 7–12 hp tractor (shown in Figure 4.1) fulfills the necessity of enabling farm mechanization and empowering the farmers. The tractor to be purchased must be compatible with the implements like cultivator, rotavator, etc. Apart from conventional agricultural applications the small tractor can also be used in transportation, running a pump using power takeoff (PTO), drive to a stationary machinery like thresher, windrower, etc. For appropriate selection of a small tractor, following few special design considerations are required:

- Introduction of a special type of spring to increase the sensitivity of the feedback system. The high hp tractors are sensitive to 15–20 kg of extra drawbar load, but smaller tractors require sensitivity to 3–6 kg of extra drawbar load.

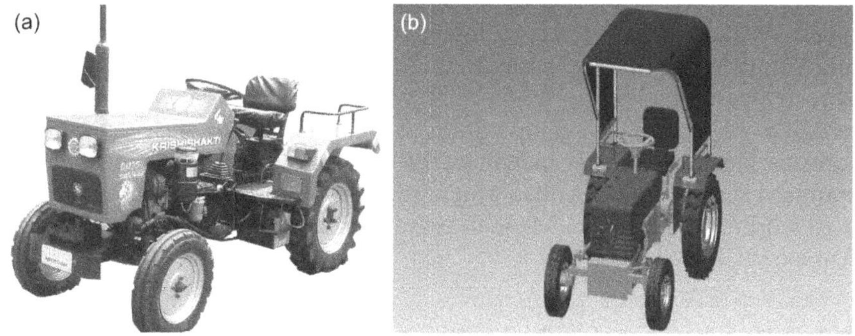

Figure 4.1 a) Krishishakti tractor (10–12 hp). b) 3D model of the compact tractor (7.5 hp).

- Mechanism to make the up and down motion of implement the smoother.
- Provision of a suitable hydraulic system.

4.3.2 Pneumatic precision planter for vegetables

Vegetables constitute about 50% share among all horticultural produce and occupy an important place in the farm sector. Mechanization of these crops can increase efficiency and cost-effectiveness. Compared to the traditional methods of transplanting the nursery-raised seedlings, vegetable seeds can be directly planted to the required plant population using a pneumatic precision planter. As it has the capability of maintaining the seeding depth (which is a critical factor for small seeds of vegetables) and planting single seeds (high singulation rate), it results in saving of "costly seeds, labor requirement and sowing time". Please see Annexure-III for more details about the design features of the planter.

4.3.3 Inter-row rotary cultivator for wide-row crops

Weeding and associated intercultural operations (shallow tilling and earthing) are tedious and time-consuming activities for the farm workers. With labor shortage, uncontrolled growth of weeds and competition for available nutrients and other inputs, the overall yield of the crop gets heavily impacted. The rotary cultivator is a perfect choice for farmers to undertake the weeding and intercultural operations. By combining the modules, it can also act as a shallow tiller for small and marginal farmers [3]. More details of the inter-row cultivator are provided in Annexure-III.

4.3.4 Offset rotavator for orchards

To perform operations like tilling, intercultural rotavators may be utilized. To perform such operation under the canopies of the trees, there is a need of offsetting and side-shifting of the tilling unit to avoid damage to canopies. As the canopy size is different for various crops, the provision of auto-adjusting the offset is required. An offset rotary tiller [4] is a PTO-operated tractor-mounted implement which is used for the pulverization of soil as secondary tillage operation as well as weeding purpose in agroforestry fields. With this machine, the farmer can avoid buying another standard rotavator for seedbed preparations as offset position locking helps it to work as a rotavator. More details of the offset rotavator are given in Annexure-III.

4.3.5 Programmable irrigation scheduler

Integrated food and water planning is essential for sustainable irrigated agriculture. There is a need to create on-farm water management for sustainable agriculture. The use of a low cost affordable irrigation scheduler can help the farmers to manage the water requirements of the crop in a sustainable and cost-effective manner. The fertilizer needs of the crop can also be taken care of by installing fertigation systems, which increases the input use efficiency of water and fertilizer. Figure 4.2 shows the scheduler connected to a field solenoid valve. The use of solar energy to operate either a submersible pump or a combination of submersible and mono-block pumps coupled with an irrigation scheduler makes this unit independent catering to all irrigation requirements of the crop. Such a system can be purchased or developed as per the schematic layout of irrigation scheduler provided in Figure 4.3. In this figure schedule 1 means setting of time, frequency and duration of watering for plant 1. Similarly, schedule 2 means setting of time, frequency and duration of watering for plant 2. Schedules may be used in

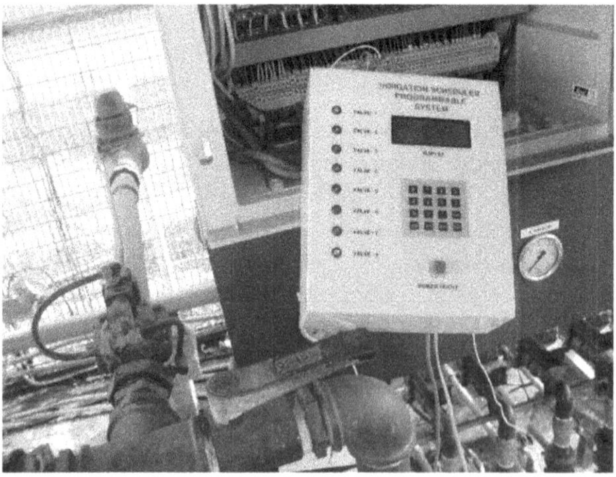

Figure 4.2 Scheduler connected to a field solenoid valve.

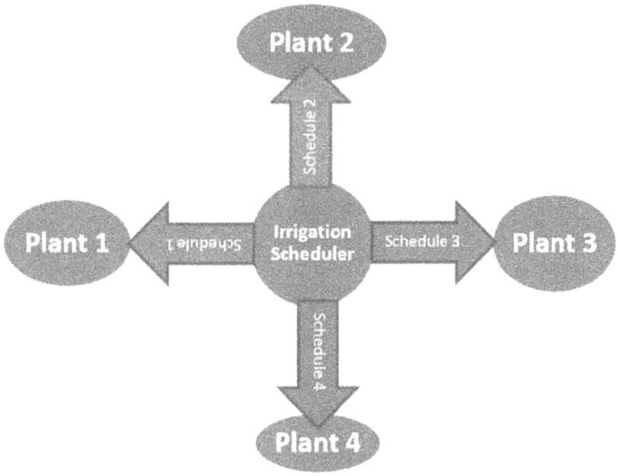

Figure 4.3 Schematic layout of an irrigation scheduler.

series or parallel arrangement. For cost-effectiveness, series arrangement such as: Schedule 1 → Schedule 2 → Schedule 4 → Schedule 3, Schedule 3 → Schedule 1 → Schedule 2, etc., is preferred.

4.3.6 Controlled atmosphere renewable (biomass/solar) energy-based stand-alone cold storage

With continuous increase in population, it is important to maximize food production per hectare of land; minimize post-harvest losses; maximize the efficiency of energy and water utilization. The horticultural crops, being of high value and more perishable, require steps in terms of post-harvest management at the first mile operations with the help of a cold room and demoisturizing facilities. The power required for those facilities can be arranged from an electricity grid, diesel generators or a stand-alone renewable energy-based system. The cold storage room utilizing solar energy and biomass energy can be used to store fresh fruits, vegetables and other perishable commodities. The solar-powered cold room enables storage of fresh produce – fruits, vegetables and flowers in the temperature range of 2°C to 8°C throughout the day. The solar panels can be mounted on the rooftop of the unit. These panels capture the available solar insulation during the sunlit day time (4–5 hours of effectively available sunlight) and the generated electricity is fed directly to the compressor via special drive systems. The schematic diagram of a vapor-compressor refrigeration system is given in Figure 4.4.

The benefits of solar cold storage systems are:

- Stand-alone operation of the unit makes it suitable for rural areas where power supply is erratic and disrupted by periodic power cuts.

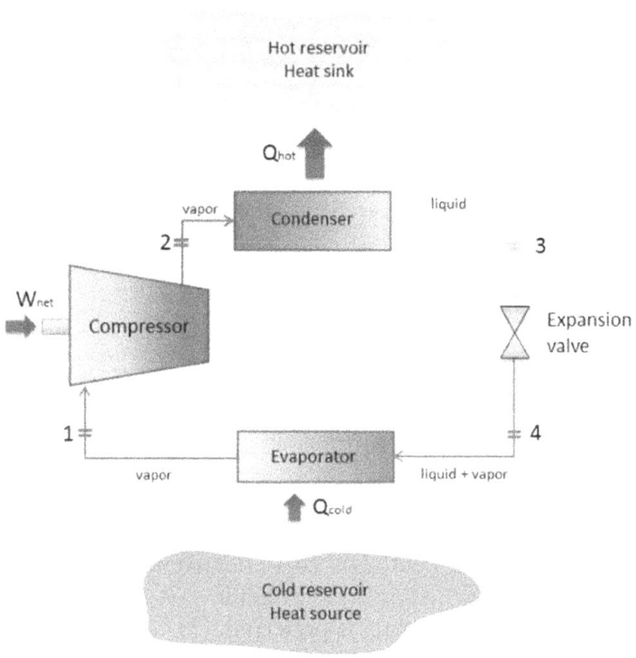

Figure 4.4 Schematic diagram of the vapor-compressor refrigeration system.

- Constant temperature as per the requirement of the fruits and vegetables to be stored in the room can be maintained which minimizes wastage of fruits and vegetables during their storage.
- Precise control of different operating parameters like RH, concentration of O_2, CO_2 and C_2H_4 to maximize the shelf-life of the stored products.

4.3.7 Ginger/turmeric processing technology: washing, slicing, drying

Ginger is one of the most attractive cash crops in a few states of India. Due to lack of proper post-harvest technology, a significant portion of crops perishes incurring a huge loss to the farmers. Thus, the farmers have no other option than to sell their crops in the local market at a very low price. The conventional way of cleaning the gingers rhizomes, slicing gingers in flakes by a manual process and subsequent solar drying in open space is not effective enough due to poor availability of sun and involvement of a lot of manual labor. Therefore, a complete post-harvest processing technology consisting of a rotary drum washer, a slicing unit, and a cabinet dryer is required [5, 6, 7]. The details of this complete unit are provided in Annexure-III.

4.3.8 Automatic biomass briquetting plant

A multifeedstock automatic briquetting machine can be developed to produce briquettes off-site from agro wastes like paddy straw, dry leaves, rice husk, grass, sawdust, etc. The complete briquetting system comprises a biomass shredding unit, a binder soaking-cum-pulverizing unit, a biomass-binder mixer, a conveyor, a hydraulically operated briquetting machine and a roller conveyor for final delivery of briquettes and a control panel. Advantages of the technology are: (a) use of multifeedstock, (b) briquette sizing as per requirement, (c) use of locally available waste material as binder, (d) 5000 briquettes per day (8h/day), (e) briquette density as per the requirement, (f) optimized shape of the briquette for better burning providing passage for free oxygen flow (honeycomb structure), (g) the same machine can be used for production of briquettes for domestic as well as industrial purpose and (h) combination of mechanical, hydraulic and electrical systems. This machine will be useful for the viable business of MSMEs and farmers. Besides, it will generate employment, save fossil fuel and reduce environmental pollution. More details of the briquetting plant are provided in Annexure-III.

4.3.9 Oil expeller technologies (1–10 TPD)

Consumption of high-quality mustard oil (Kachi Ghani grade) is highly prevalent due to its medicinal and preservation characteristics. A series of mechanical oil expellers (Figure 4.5) for marginal-small farmers are available to expel the desired percentage of oil before the oil cake is fed to the solvent extraction plant. It has the benefits of less operating cost, extra recovery and less manpower requirement. The pungent oil can be extracted around 0.4% (average of four pressings) and the residue oil cake around 10%, due to optimized parameters like moisture, temperature, compression ratios and residence time for the completion of enzymatic action to produce better pungent oil and cake [8]. Some of the features of oil expellers are:

- Water-cooled chambers to keep the temperature of oil and cake under control for extraction of better-quality pungent oil.
- In-built enclosed cake conveying system for recycling of the cake which protects the pungency from evaporation.
- Improved the life cycle of fast wearing components through design and better materials.

4.3.10 Fully automatic biodiesel plant

The available economic feedstocks in the market for production of biodiesel are mainly animal tallow, fatty acid distillates, stearin, acid oil, used cooking oil, etc. To produce biodiesel from any feedstock having such diverse

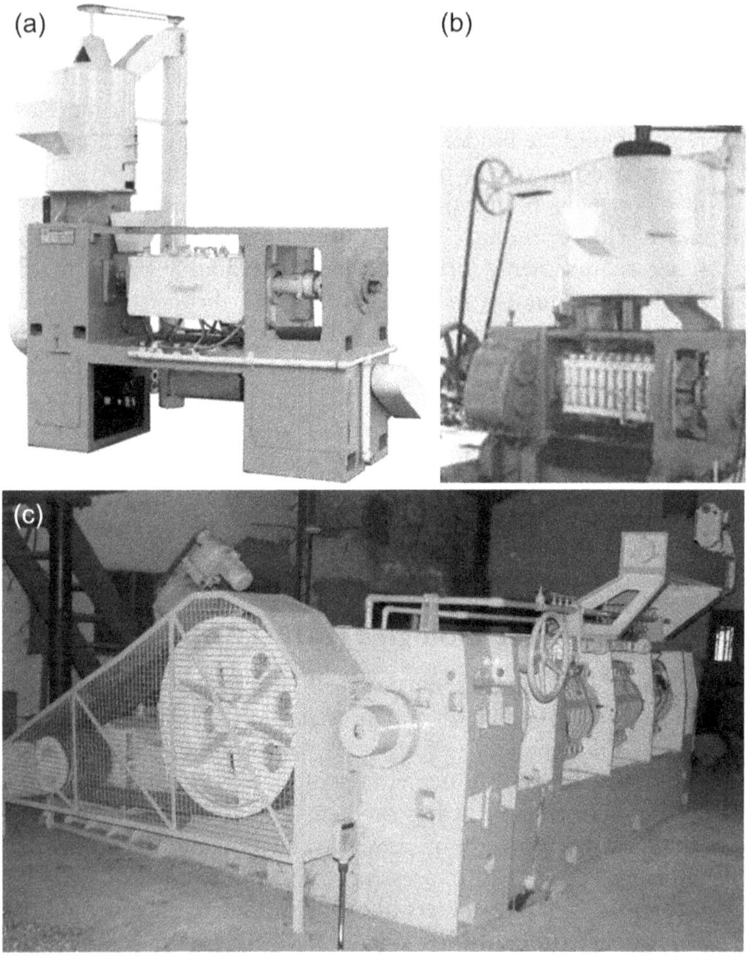

Figure 4.5 a) 1 TPD oil expeller. b) 6 TPD oil expeller. c) 10 TPD oil expeller.

free fatty acid (FFA) percentage requires a fully automated plant. The fully automated biodiesel plant needs programmable logic controller (PLC) and human machine interface (HMI)-based systems, hence requires minimum manual intervention. It has added features such as methanol recovery, degumming and glycerolysis for a better-quality diesel output. The feedstock for the plant is any type of oil/fat with (0 to 100 % FFA) to reduce dependence on Jatropha and other tree-borne oilseeds (TBOs) and rather use cost-effective alternatives through processing of waste products such as animal fat, acid oil, fatty acid distillates, etc. This plant gives the unique solution to handle these feedstocks. The maximum automation of the plant ensures a cost-effective production line and increase in productivity. The processing cost per liter of biodiesel in such plants ranges from Rs. 7 to Rs. 12 only excluding feedstock cost. It has become possible to produce biodiesel at less than Rs. 40 per liter using this plant. Hence, manufacturers/farmers may find it a very attractive business model as the selling point. The process parameters of biodiesel production from animal fat, tung, Jatropha oil, karanj, fatty acid distillate, mahua oil, acid oil and waste cooking oil (WCO) have been optimized. **Table 4.1** shows optimization of the lab-scale biodiesel production from different feedstocks [9]. In all processes, preheating temperature and reaction temperature have been maintained at 60°C. The settling time has been kept as 4 hours. To recover methanol temperature as 70°C and vacuum in the range of 350–400 mmHg has been maintained. The plant consists of a feedstock reservoir, a preheating tank, a methanol reservoir, a methoxide tank, a reactor tank, a methanol recovery unit, settling tanks and a glycerolysis unit. Automation of the biodiesel plant is achieved by integrating the temperature sensors, flow meter solenoid valves, level sensors, motors, pumps and heaters through a PLC. The degree of automation has been developed to eliminate manual intervention to the extent possible. The whole automation process is easily managed with the HMI. The plant creates an opportunity of employment generation starting from feedstock collection, biodiesel production, quality check, transportation, selling of glycerol (byproduct) and biodiesel. One single plant can generate employment for up to ten people.

4.3.11 Solar biomass and electric powered hybrid dryer

Shelf-life of most of the agricultural products can be extended by regulating moisture content. Moisture creates reactions and reproduction of microorganisms, resulting in decay of agricultural products. The excess of moisture can be reduced through appropriate drying methods. Open sun drying is the most widespread conventional method for food preservation. The major disadvantage of this technique is dust, insects, rodents, pathogens, microorganisms and other animals infest the food materials which seriously degrades the food quality thereby resulting in a negative trade potential with lowered economic returns. In addition, this drying method also requires labor and long drying time (2–3 days). There is a need for efficient and affordable drying methods. Varieties of electrical energy driven dryers are available but become uneconomical due to high energy cost and remain unaffordable for farmers. Therefore, low cost and locally manufactured solar dryers may be emphasized.

Other than solar, biomass is a renewable energy resource available in abundance in various rural areas. Combustion of biomass in the presence of excess air in a combustor liberates heat energy, inert gases and ash. A cross counter flow heat exchanger removes the heat from the combustion gases

Table 4.1 Optimization of the lab-scale biodiesel production from different feedstocks

	Optimized parameters							
Optimizing parameter	*Tung seed oil*	*Jatropha oil*	*Animal fat*	*Mahua oil (after esterification)*	*Karanj oil*	*Acid oil (after glycerolysis)*	*Fatty acid distillate (after glycerolysis)*	*Used cooking oil*
Molar ratio (methanol:oil)	5:1	5:1	7.5:1	8:1	6:1	6.2:1	6.2:1	5:1
Methanol used (v/w) (methanol/oil)	20%	20%	30%	32.32% (~32%)	24.2 % (~24%)	25.25% (~25%)	25.25% (~25%)	20%
Methanol used (w/w) (methanol/oil)	16%	16%	24%	25.6% (~26%)	19.2% (~19%)	20%	20%	16%
Catalyst (KOH) concentration	2.0%	3.0%	2.5%	3.0%	2.5%	2.5%	2.5%	2.5%
Reaction time (minutes)	30 min	30 min	90 min	45 min	40 min	60 min	60 min	60 min
For 170 L batch								
Feedstock (average density of oil 0.9 g/mL)	170 L 153 kg	170 L 153 kg	170 L 153 kg	170 L 153 kg	170 L 153 kg	170 L 153 kg	170 L 153 kg	170 L 153 kg
Molar ratio (methanol:oil)	5:1	5:1	7.5:1	8:1	6:1	6.2:1	6.2:1	5:1
Methanol (v/v) (methanol/oil)	30 L	30 L	46 L	49 L	37 L	38.25 L	38.25 L	30 L
Catalyst (KOH) (w/v)	2.0% 3.06 kg	3.0% 4.59 kg	2.5% 3.825 kg	3.0% 4.59 kg	2.5% 3.825 kg	2.5% 3.825 kg	2.5% 3.825 kg	2.5% 3.825 kg

and exchanges with the air circulated in the drying chamber for drying the material.

4.3.12 Biogas from grass/weeds, etc.

Biomass from grassland is suitable for producing biogas. Biogas at present occupies a smaller percentage in the energy generation scenario. Energy recovery from biogas by anaerobic digestion (AD) utilizing sewage sludge, recirculated slurry and other animal dung has been well known for several decades. However, the use of biomass residues or grasses for production of biogas has started recently. Perennial grasses are ideal feedstock for renewable energy production due to their high potential of dry matter yields, fast growth and higher biomass yield. The methane yield depends on the time of harvest and its biodegradability. If the harvest is done after a longer growing period, it will lead to higher lignin content in grasses, thereby causing slower biodegradation and lower methane yield. Production of biogas from grassland can not only guarantee high greenhouse gas savings, but it can also contribute to economic growth, employment generation through the use of the byproducts like slurry which can be converted to value-added products like manure, briquettes, a substrate for incense stick making and overall energy safety.

4.4 EMERGING TECHNOLOGIES AND NEW INNOVATIONS IN AGRICULTURE

The agriculture sector is going through various challenges such as shortage of labor, depletion of natural resources, i.e., water, and degradation of soil quality due to excessive usage of fertilizers and pesticides. The world is moving at a rapid pace to adopt modern technologies in agriculture to save natural resources using optimum input. The level of farm mechanization varies through different stages of the crop cycle [10].

With emerging technologies, there is a need for modern machinery for rice and wheat crops starting from seedbed preparation to harvesting, increasing the crop productivity by reducing direct labor involvement and improving the farmer's economic and social conditions. A few of the emerging technologies to revamp agriculture in the coming years are described below:

Electric tractors and power tillers: Electric tractors and power tillers can be better alternatives to existing tractors because of the less operation cost, reduced noise, vibration and harshness (NVH) and significant reduction in the environmental pollution. The tractor consists of an electric drive system having a transmission unit and a battery-operated powered system. In an electric tractor, the highest cost component will be the battery. Therefore, a machine variant which will run on battery continuously for one hour is proposed. But this requires a facility for frequent charging, and lack of charging infrastructure is the major concern for acceptance of electric tractors and power tillers.

Innovative solar charging systems can play a pivotal role in this regard. A solar tree, a space-rationalized, minimum shadow generating and efficient solar-based technology, can be the solution. The electric tractor and power tiller can be plugged onto a solar tree to charge batteries. These electric vehicles will reduce operational cost to the farmers as diesel prices are increasing day by day. This form of renewable energy can be used for powering first generation e-tractors and e-power tillers to curtail the expenditure related to price-volatile fossil fuels. This will help curb millions of tons of CO_2 and other greenhouse gas (GHG) emissions across the globe. Besides, the surplus energy generated can be fed into energy grids for surplus trading. This surplus power trading will help the farmers attain a certain degree of income consistency in the very uncertain climate-linked agricultural activities.

Artificial intelligence (AI) and Internet of things (IoT): Artificial intelligence-powered IoT platforms can be used to help the farmers in getting real-time data of their crops and acting accordingly to protect crops having better nutrition [11]. These kinds of initiatives will help farmers to transform the insights from the collected data into farm-specific, crop-specific actionable advisories via mobile in vernacular languages [11].

Use of drones, global positioning system (GPS), geographic information system (GIS) and satellite-based technologies: To meet the challenges of sustainability and maintaining demand in the agricultural sector, start-ups like Pigeonis are providing [12] efficient drone solutions for agriculture services and spraying. The drones are equipped with highly sensitive cameras and near infrared (NIR) sensors that collect high-quality data. The data can be further used for monitoring plant health, harvesting and managing crops in better ways. This helps in increasing yields by using resources effectively.

Big data sectors are used to improve crop traceability and sustainability. For this, start-ups like Cropin [13] use a suite of software and mobile apps powered by GIS and data science to deliver a range of services to farmers. There are also start-ups like Oxen that utilize satellite imagery and big data to analyze crop life cycle. Crop data is captured using mobile-enabled solutions. This data can be used to assist the farmer in making informed decisions such as which crop will be right for that land at that season.

A number of technologies, presented in previous paragraphs, can improve the level of farm mechanization. These implements and technologies cover a various range of applications throughout the crop cycle. A number of R&D institutions are working on various technologies focusing on precision agriculture which will further enhance farm mechanization and crop productivity.

4.5 DIGITIZATION AND IT IN AGRICULTURE

In the present environment, traditional knowledgebase may not be sufficient for the enhancement of the produce quality due to dynamic change in ecological conditions, adverse effect of agrochemicals viz. pesticides/fertilizers on the soil fertility, development of resistance against the use of such external measure and their impact on the environment. These situations can also be handled efficiently by the use of artificial intelligence and data analytics technologies in the agricultural sector. The unpredictable weather conditions, food security challenges, continuous demand of enhancement in the farm productivity, require "smart agriculture" for the benefits of both farmers and consumers. The "smart agriculture", as sometimes referred as Agriculture 4.0, encompasses the use of information and communication technologies (ICTs), artificial intelligence (AI), Internet of things (IoT), ubiquitous data gathering in digital form, data analytics, ultra-low altitude drones backed up with on-ground automation, etc. for appropriate decision-making and timely response. ICT and digitization help the farmers to become aware of upcoming scientific development, how to reduce the cost of production, use the resources with maximum efficiency, especially the power and water for better productivity. Furthermore, information like advanced knowledge of soil fertility and measures against the predicted hazards of crop disease as well as infestation of pests are some other areas where data analytics and information platforms can be of use. IoT technologies, if implemented in agricultural farms, alone can give various insights to the farmers about microclimatic conditions, different kinds of stresses in crops and probable infestation of pests and diseases which can adversely affect the final produce. An Internet-connected multipurpose e-kiosk system, useful for smart agriculture, can be installed in various farms.

GYAN (interface for Greater Yield with Agricultural kNowledge) fills up the information gap between the researchers, agricultural scientists and farmers. The said e-kiosk system has a user-friendly multilingual touch screen interface that can provide suitable and decentralized solutions for the rural sector. The developed system is designed to run on solar as well as grid power and can be deployed at panchayat buildings, block offices, community centers, etc. to disseminate information in local languages in the remote and far-flung rural areas. As depicted in Figure 4.6, GYAN e-kiosk is envisioned to interface with the IoT nodes in the farms of different farmers without any need of separately managing a computational infrastructure for the collection of real-time data from different fields. The e-Kiosk

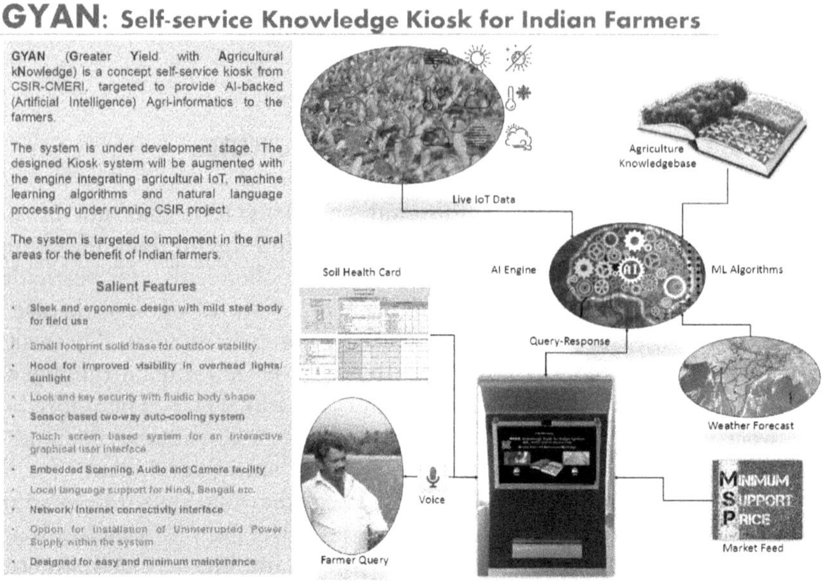

Figure 4.6 GYAN e-kiosk with backend technological suits for agricultural application.

is supposed to be connected with the backend cloud system equipped with different AI models and data analytics platforms, which uses real-time IoT datasets and soil data using soil health cards for providing recommendations to the farmers. While making recommendations, weather forecasts for the geographical regions along with historical dataset and agricultural knowledgebase for different crops can also be taken into account.

Further to the above, a cloud-based IoT platform is also needed for collecting real-time dataset from the node deployed in agricultural farms spanning across the geographical regions. This IoT cloud platform can further be used for deployment of machine learning models and perform data analytics for pushing different recommendations to the farmers. For this purpose, CSIR-CMERI developed an IoT cloud platform "SAGITA".

BIBLIOGRAPHY

1. Department of Agriculture, Cooperation & Farmers Welfare, Government of India. *Agriculture Annual Report 2018–19.* Report is published by Department of Agriculture, Cooperation and Farmers Welfare, Ministry of Agriculture & Farmers Welfare. http://agricoop.nic.in/annual-report, 2018-2019
2. https://www.fao.org/family-farming/detail/en/c/459197/, 2022
3. *Design & Development of Tractor Mounted Inter-row Rotary Cultivator for Wide Row Crops*, funded by SERB, DST, Principal Investigator and

Co-Investigator: Dr. Baldev Dogra, Research Engineer, PAU, Ludhiana and Mr. Jagdish M, Scientist, CSIR-CMERI CoEFM, Ludhiana, 2018.

4. *Design & Development of Offset Rotavator for Orchards*, funded by SERB, DST, Principal Investigator and Co-Investigator: Dr. Baldev Dogra, Research Engineer, PAU, Ludhiana, Dr. R. N. Pateriya, Professor, GBPUA&T, Pantnagar and Mr. Jagdish M, Scientist, CSIR-CMERI CoEFM, Ludhiana, 2018.
5. C. Loha, A. Chatterjee, L.G. Das, B. Chakarborty, and P.K. Chatterjee. Ginger drying machine. Design Registration No.: 297172, 2017.
6. K.K. Mistry, C. Loha, A. Ganguly, and H. Hirani. Continuous moisture measurement and monitoring system for ginger dryer. Copyright Applied, 2020.
7. L.G. Das, C. Loha, P.K. Chatterjee, R.K. Padhi, and S. Mukherjee. Ginger slicing machine. Design Registration No.: 294632, 2017.
8. CSIR-CMERI. *Design & Development of 6 TPD Oil Expeller for Achieving Pungency in Oil from Mustard Seed*, Project No. SSP023812 and *Fabrication 50 TPD Modern Oil Expeller*, Project No. GAP-022612, 2019.
9. Krishnendu Kundu, Prabhu Dutt Sharma, Jetinder Raturi, Pradeep Rajan, and Harish Hirani. 1TDP fully automatic biodiesel plant: fully automatic biodiesel plant. Design Registration, CMERI Ref. CSIR-CMERI/IPMG/DR/2020–21/57, 2020.
10. https://yourstory.com/2018/02/iot-big-data-equipment-farmers-agri-startups?utm_pageloadtype=scroll, 2022
11. https://fasal.co/, 2022
12. https://pigeonis.in/, 2022
13. https://www.cropin.com/, 2022

Chapter 5

Manufacturing and automation as a recovery path toward sustainable growth

Manufacturing is vital for coping with the crisis, enhancing employability and reducing overall poverty. To spread manufacturing as a viable source of income, it becomes essential to integrate manufacturing with innovation.

5.1 INTRODUCTION

One or two innovative manufacturing technologies will not solve the country's economic problems, but perhaps a revitalization of the entire enterprise and ecosystem with a dedicated and robust logistical (transport, power, supply chain) grid is required. This can only be achieved by involving micro and small enterprises, which provide jobs to millions of people, by helping them in developing innovative manufacturing processes. In short, developing affordable innovative manufacturing machines are vital to increase the employability.

Various high end computer numerical control (CNC) machines, 3D printing machines, advanced computer-aided design (CAD)/computer-aided manufacturing (CAM) software, heat treatment processes, coating and plating technologies are available in academic and research institutions. Such institutions disseminate knowledgebase to the potential young minds through formal education or skill development programs. In addition, if the infrastructure and humongous R&D knowledgebase of those institutions are shared with the micro, small and medium enterprises (MSMEs) and start-ups at nominal rates, it might give a tremendous boost to manufacturing productivities of those enterprises. Few companies may become aggressive, successful in changing manufacturing practices and achieve significant improvements in productivity and reduce product defects.

Apart from sharing infrastructure and knowledgebase, the public funded institutes can launch the conceptual ideas into the real world by transferring technologies to MSMEs and become technology accelerators by providing engineering services to the industries. In other words, public-funded research institutions can sign agreements with a number of manufacturing partners to change technology from a low volume, proof-of-concept phase to commercial large-volume production so that industries can earn profit

DOI: 10.1201/9781003331179-5

and improve economics. Collectively, this creates a sustainable ecosystem of high-mix manufacturing primarily to demonstrate how quickly MSMEs can deliver exactly what their customers want. Such interaction between industries and R&D institutions will provide win-win solutions. The R&D laboratories can start researching to tap existing resources of industries and improve those by following a model of lean implementation, empowering workers to minimize cost, improve quality and provide more flexibility in manufacturing. In other words, government-funded R&D institutions may focus on the development and applications (time-bound translation of advanced/innovative research into real-life technologies) required by MSMEs and on benefitting the maximum number of people from them.

Apart from manufacturing technologies, effective implementation is going to play a key role in productivity. Special emphasis must be given to minimize/recycle the waste generated during the manufacturing process such as scraps, overruns, trims and other processing wastes (i.e., misprinted or defective products). Therefore, a scheme must be drawn to explain the essential components of and growth opportunities for innovative manufacturing in strengthening the country's economy. Requirement of lowering costs, greater precision and multi-utilities from components/systems will inevitably lead to greater innovation and excellence. It is preferable to count the time required for manufacturing the components and the time required to make complete assembly of those components. Such counting of time provides information to reduce the manufacturing time. It is important to understand that to spread such knowledge/education across the nation (including villages, towns), the universities must form new skill development programs in collaboration with the industries to strengthen manufacturing and innovation to guide students to meet the new challenges in manufacturing, design, business innovation and product realization. Extensive and thorough workers' training and empowerment in the decision-making are essential to fulfill/serve various national technical and non-technical projects and create/develop products/processes for common people. With those projects, students will have an understanding of national problems, work experience in manufacturing machines and learn creative methods to solve the problems. For this kind of ecosystem, government funding, willingness, students' fellowships and visionary leadership are essential.

5.2 WHAT IS TO BE LEARNED IN MANUFACTURING PROCESSES?

The manufacturing techniques are divided into three categories, namely, formative manufacturing (injection molding, casting, stamping and forging), subtractive manufacturing (CNC, turning and drilling) and additive manufacturing (3D printing). A number of micro and small manufacturing enterprises utilize conventional manufacturing processes (i.e., machining, welding and metal casting), manual manufacturing techniques, and remain unaware of new-scientific "manufacturing technologies". Majority of the workers employed in the micro and small enterprises (MSEs) do not have formal training in the manufacturing processes and stay ignorant of standard operating practices. They acquire the knowledge through on-the-job training by working along with their seniors for long duration and find difficulty to innovate to improve the product quality. In this section, manufacturing practices and common mistakes related to machining, welding [1] and metal casting are described.

5.2.1 Machining practices and issues

Machining is a manufacturing (turning, milling, drilling, shaping, boring, grinding, broaching, etc.) process to produce the desired shape and size by removing the excess material (metal, plastics, woods, ceramics, etc.) from a preformed blank. A cutting tool is used to remove the excess material by shearing action. The cutting tool can be classified into two groups. (a) Single point cutting tools (e.g., turning tools, drills, etc.) and (b) multi-point cutting tools (e.g., milling cutters, broaching tools, etc.).

5.2.1.1 Turning practices and issues

A lathe machine is a versatile machine and it is available in almost every workshop. Turning operation performed on a lathe machine is the subtraction of material from the surface of a rotating cylindrical workpiece to reduce the diameter to the desirable dimension having a smooth metallic finish. Annexure-IV highlights common mistakes made during turning operation, which unnecessarily increases the material wastage. Those mistakes must be avoided.

5.2.1.2 Milling practices and issues

It is a process performed with a rotating cutter to subtract the material from a rectangular/square bar. Unlike the lathe machine, where the workpiece is rotated against the tool, a milling cutter spins against the workpiece. Important steps to be followed to avoid any mistake during milling operation are detailed in Annexure-IV.

5.2.1.3 Drilling practices and issues

Drilling is a very common cutting process to produce holes of circular cross-sections in a solid material. More information on the essential steps required for the drilling operations, the need of indentation, operations after drilling, surface finish, selection of cutting parameters and the type of tools needed for carrying out those operations are discussed in Annexure-IV.

5.2.1.4 Most common mistakes during machining operations

- **Not following the geometrical dimensioning and tolerances (GD&T) guidelines:** Most of the operators working in micro/small enterprises are unaware about geometrical dimensioning and tolerances (GD&T) and its related manufacturing cost, which is a function of deviation (i.e., dimensional tolerances, geometric tolerances) from true geometry. Due to this, deviations in the component dimensions occur requiring rectifications/rejection. In view of this, there is a need to provide skill development on how to read and understand the drawings and teach them the importance of producing quality products so that the mistakes can be minimized. Figure 5.1 provides the basic information regarding GD&T.

  The left side picture explains the drawing symbols like straightness, flatness, perpendicular and concentricity, etc., to guide the operator to understand how to machine the components accurately to achieve the desired quality requirements and based on this understanding how to select the suitable cutting tools and operational sequences to follow during machining processes. Similarly, the picture on the right side gives a clear idea about types of fitting needed between the two assembly parts for properly fitting in the assembly and to produce the desired results. For example, in the first case the requirement is to produce a loose running fit for the mating shaft and the hole and to achieve that a fit operator has to produce the hole size to meet the dimensional tolerances as per the H11 standard. Similarly, the corresponding shaft is to be manufactured to meet the c11 tolerance standard. In this case just after reading the drawing requirements, the operator notes down the tolerance values as per the standard chart and selects the tools, machines, measuring instruments and operation sequences to achieve

Types of Tolerance	Geometric Characteristic	Symbol
Form	Straightness	⏤
	Flatness	⏥
	Circularity	○
	Cylindricity	⌭
Orientation	Perpendicularity	⊥
	Angularity	∠
	Parallelism	//
Location	Positional	⌖
	Concentricity	◎
	Symmetry	⌯
Runout	Circular Runout	↗
	Total Runout	⌰
Profile	Profile of a line	⌒
	Profile of a surface	⌓

Types of Fit	Hole	Shaft
Loose Running Fit:- Suitable for loose pulleys and the looser fastener fits where freedom of assembly is of prime importance.	H11	c11
Free Running Fit:- Where accuracy is not essential, but good for large temperature variation,high running speeds,heavy journal pressures	H9	d10
Close Running Fit:- Suitable for lubricated bearing, greater accuracy, accurate location, where no substantial temperature difference is encountered.	H8	f7
Sliding Fits:- Suitable for precision location fits. Shafts are expensive to manufacture since the clearances are small and they are not recommended for running fits except in precision equipment where the shaft loadings are very light.	H7	g6
Lecatianal Clearance Fits:- Provides snug fit for locating stationary parts; but can be freely assembled and disassembled.	H7	h6

Figure 5.1 Basic information about GD&T.

the desired quality requirements. Similarly, depending upon the type of fitting requirements, an operator follows the standard procedures to produce the quality products.

To summarize, there is a need to understand that there are three types of fits: "clearance fit: tolerance zone of the hole > the tolerance zone of the shaft", "interference fit: tolerance zone of the hole < the tolerance zone of the shaft" and "transition fit: tolerance zone of the hole ≈ the tolerance zone of the shaft". For shafts, base tolerance grades are "a" to "z", where "a" to "h" is for clearance fit, "js" to "n" for transition fit and "p" to "z" for interference fit. For holes, the letters are in capital.

- **Mistakes in using measuring instruments:** Some precautionary measures are taken while using the measuring instruments as there are possibilities of deviations. Mistakes can be controlled/eliminated by taking the following precautionary measures:
  1. Parallax error (refer Figure 5.2): This error occurs when one observes the object from an angle, which leads to erroneous reading. In order to eliminate this error, the operator should take the measurement reading by positioning eyes directly above the scale. This error is quite common in smaller machine shops where conventional types of measuring instruments like plain vernier caliper, plain micrometer, screw gauge, etc. are used. This kind of error can be avoided by using digital types of measuring instruments, displaying reading in discrete numerals.
  2. It is always important to take all the readings in the same unit system during the measurement (i.e., MKS/CGS/FPS). In many cases during reverse engineering or adopting drawings from different sources measurements may be in different unit systems, then it should be immediately converted to the appropriate unit system.

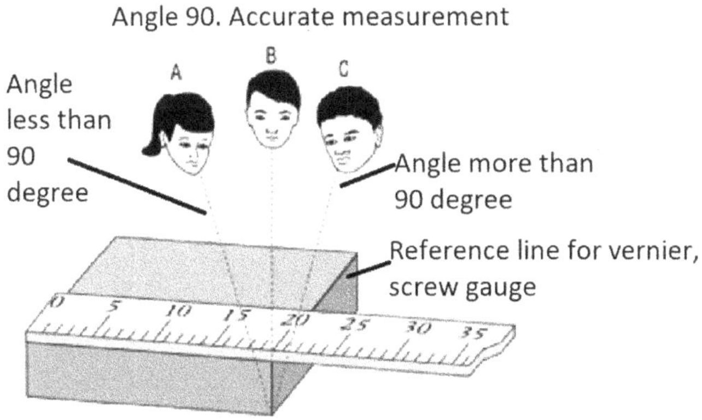

Figure 5.2 Possibilities of error in reading the measuring instruments.

Otherwise, the two different components produced by using two separate measuring systems (MKS/CGS) will be unsuitable to meet the assembly requirements and finally one may have to re-produce the parts to achieve the desired accuracy that will incur the losses to the machine shop in terms of time, manpower, machine and also wastage of material.

3. A common mistake is assumption of getting better readings of the measurements by applying excessive force on the jaws of the measuring instruments like, vernier caliper or micrometer screw gauge. But it is not true as it is always better to apply a gentle force on the jaws of the instruments while taking the readings to get better readings of the measurement. One can practically experience the effect of excessive force while taking the readings on some components like thin sheets and wires which are easily deformable. As applying excessive pressure on the measuring instruments not only may damage the fragile components and can also cause errors in measurements, it can also damage the precision edges of the measuring instruments which are costlier and not procured on a regular basis.
4. The instruments, to be used for the measurement, should not have any zero error. Cross checking of zero error on the instruments can be easily done by bringing both the jaws of the caliper in contact with each other (in case of a vernier caliper). The zero markings on both the vernier scale and the main scale should align at this point (Figure 5.3). If the zero markings on both vernier and main scales are properly aligned then there will be no zero error on the instrument if not then there is a zero error and the appropriate corrections should be applied during each measurement either by adding or subtracting the amount of error from the measured dimensions (depending upon the nature of error, i.e., positive or negative). In the case of a micrometer, one should move the spindle of the micrometer until it touches the anvil. If the zero mark on the thimble is not aligned with the zero of the datum line of sleeve, the micrometer is said to have zero error. If the micrometer reads plus, it has a *minus zero error*. The error will have to be subtracted from the actual reading. If the micrometer reads minus, it has the *plus*

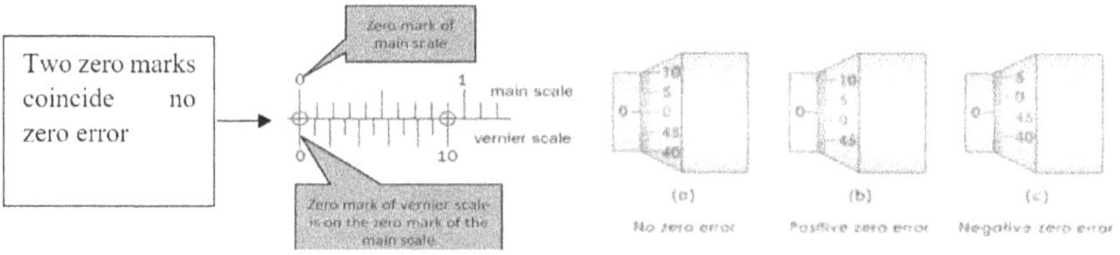

Figure 5.3 Cross checking of zero errors.

zero error. The error will have to be added to the actual reading. Zero error can be removed from a micrometer by adjusting the barrel with the "C" spanner available in the micrometer box.

All the dimensions which are measured without compensating the zero error will produce a component with dimensional errors and may cause the rejection of the component if the error value is beyond the tolerance limit.

5. An operator should always ensure that the surfaces of the object, to be measured, are properly cleaned and dried before the start of the measurement to get an error free reading in a measurement. As the presence of any foreign material in between the part to be measured and the measuring instruments will give a false reading and that false readings may continue to affect measurement of many more components as long as that foreign material is sticking to the instrument.
6. One common mistake of operators is keeping the instruments after their use without checking whether the jaws of the caliper or spindle and anvil of the micrometer screw gauge are closed or have some gap between them. Presence of any dirt on the measurement surfaces while closing the gauge will damage the measuring surfaces by grinding of the dirt in between the two surfaces. As a standard practice, the following procedure is used for storing the measuring instruments for the enhancement of their usage life and also to get accurate readings every time:
   - Avoid storing the measuring instruments in direct sunlight.
   - Store the instruments in a ventilated place with low humidity.
   - Store the instruments in a place where less or no dust is present.
   - Store the instruments in a case/container, which should not be kept on the floor.
   - When storing the instruments like vernier caliper/micrometer, always leave a gap of 0.1–1.0 mm between the measuring faces.
   - Do not store the measuring instruments in a clamped state.
7. Over-tightening the thimble of a micrometer screw gauge is one of the most common mistakes. It is always advisable to apply a gentle pressure to avoid damage to both the instrument and the component being measured.
8. Thread gauges are manufactured with special materials with precision machining and many after-treatment processes as they play a very important role in deciding the type of threads on the object to be measured. These gauges need to be handled carefully and stored in a controlled temperature environment as these instruments are very sensitive toward the variation in temperature. It is also very important to make best efforts to store the precision gauges in a place with as little humidity as possible to prevent instruments from being rusted and ruining the quality of their performance.

9. Suitable lubrication oil should be applied periodically to avoid rusting, and accuracy of the instruments should be tracked regularly, and more importantly, operators should be trained to use them.
10. As in a machine shop several types of instruments are used and each type requires a specific procedure to be followed to enhance their usages, adequate training of the concerned operators plays a very important role in maintaining the instrument's accuracy for a longer period of time and also reduces the recurring cost involved in frequent procuring of these costly instruments.

- **Selection of jobs which are not profitable:** It is a known fact that everyone cannot do everything. Choices should be made wisely after analyzing the number of changes needed to take the new task and deciding whether the new task becomes a strength or weakness in the long run, etc. Hence choice of jobs must be made carefully based on the merits and demerits. It is very important for a machine shop to know its strengths and weaknesses in terms of both infrastructure facility and knowledge level of the manpower and their ability to adapt to the dynamic changes in the market requirements.

5.2.2 Welding practice and issues

The construction and manufacturing projects require some form of welding, from assembly production to maintenance/repair. The automotive sector is one the largest user of welding, but finding a skilled and experienced welder is not that easy. Figure 5.4 indicates the enormous scope of welding

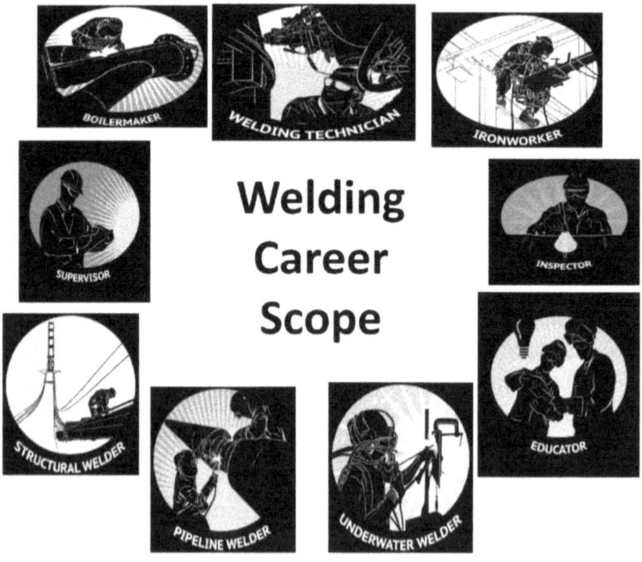

Figure 5.4 Scope of welding as a career.

as a career. Even though an arc welding machine is commonly available with micro and small enterprises, for appropriate outputs, there is a need to understand this process with scientific temper.

5.2.2.1 Essential requirements for good arc welding

For correct welding practice, the five major factors: "correct electrode size", "correct current", "correct arc length", "correct travel speed" and "correct electrode angle" are expected to be established. Determination of correct electrode size is dictated by the joint location and edge preparation. The arc length being too long/short is harmful from a welding point of view. A long arc increases the volume of the molten metal and too short arcs do not adequately melt the base metal. Furthermore, correct speed is essential to avoid impurities, gas bubbles, metal pile up. In filet/deep-groove welding, the electrode angle is of significance. In general, when performing a filet weld, the electrode shall be positioned perpendicular to the weld line and bisect the angle between the plates (as shown in Figure 5.5). When there is an undercut in a structural member, the angle of the arc is reduced and the arc is diverted toward the member.

5.2.2.2 Common arc welding mistakes

Even with the right selection of electrode, current and position, there are possibilities of quality compromises such as: "porous weld", "undercut" "distortion", "inclusion". These kinds of problems occur due to an unclean surface, wet, unclean or damaged electrode, faulty joint preparation, incomplete slag removal between passes, improper setup and fixture, etc. Compliance with the following guidelines may ensure quality welding:

i. Ensure the complete cleanliness of the joint interface and the electrode. The joint should be free from any paint, grease, oil, moisture, foreign materials, etc.

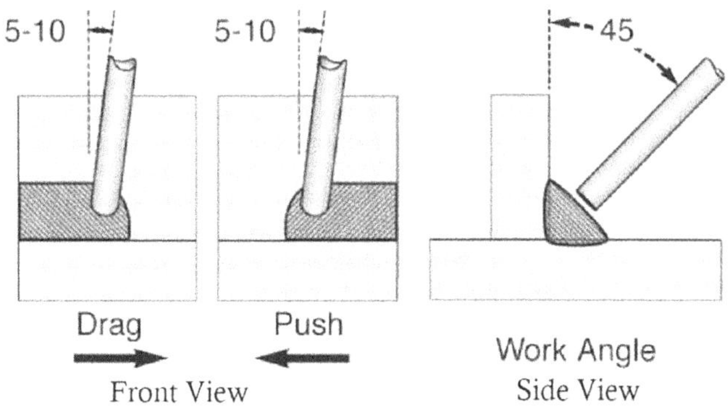

Figure 5.5 Electrode angles for correct welding practice.

ii. Preheat the base metal if required to ensure the temperature requirements are met.
iii. Ensure no crack or uneven surface is present in the base material.
iv. Special care must be taken for fillet and groove welding.
v. Inspect welding work continuously and repair any defective weld immediately. Overlaps and undercuts must be properly repaired.
vi. Ensure smoothness of the finished weld surface.

5.2.2.3 Welding of cast iron

When welding cast iron the following items must be evaluated, regardless of the type of iron being welded, or the process/equipment/electrode/filler metal being used, to avoid large stress-induced cracking:

Base metal preparation [2]: Clean base metal without any casting tear/porosity/shrinkage defects/inclusions is a prima facie requirement. In case of any defect, it should be addressed before the welding operation. Similarly, casting shells, surface coating, sand, rust, paint, oil, grease, moisture, dirt, etc. are to be removed prior to welding; otherwise, weld non-linearities may occur. Oil and grease may be removed by heating the substrate at temperatures ranging from 370°C to 480°C. Casted parts such as submersible pump casings often are impregnated with silts, deposits or sand, to be cleaned by polishing the cast surface until it become free of defects.

Joint design [3, 4]*:* Single-V or single-U groove welds are required in thin cast iron. Standard steel weld grooves are acceptable for shallow repairs using steel filler metals. Groove angles should be increased when using nickel base filler metals to allow for manipulation of the stagnant weld pool. Because nickel base electrodes achieve less root penetration than steel electrodes, the root face must be reduced. Grooves should be used for thicknesses greater than about 1/2 in. (12.7 mm) to evenly distribute the stresses induced during welding. When both sides of the joint are accessible, double welded joints are effective in such applications. A double V-groove or a double bevel groove should be used for thicknesses up to 3/4 in. (19 mm). A double U-groove or double J-groove should be considered for thicknesses greater than 3/4 in. A modified U-groove may be used when only one side of the section is accessible. This allows access to the joint root and reduces the width of the weld face, reducing both weld metal mass and shrinkage stresses caused by shrinkage (Figure 5.6). When welding a thick base metal, the groove faces are frequently buttered. In this manner, the initial welding on the low ductility cast iron is done with less residual stress.

Heat input: The size of a weld's heat affected zone (HAZ) is determined by the heat input. As a result, lower heat input processes are best suited for welding cast iron. Welding currents should be kept to a bare

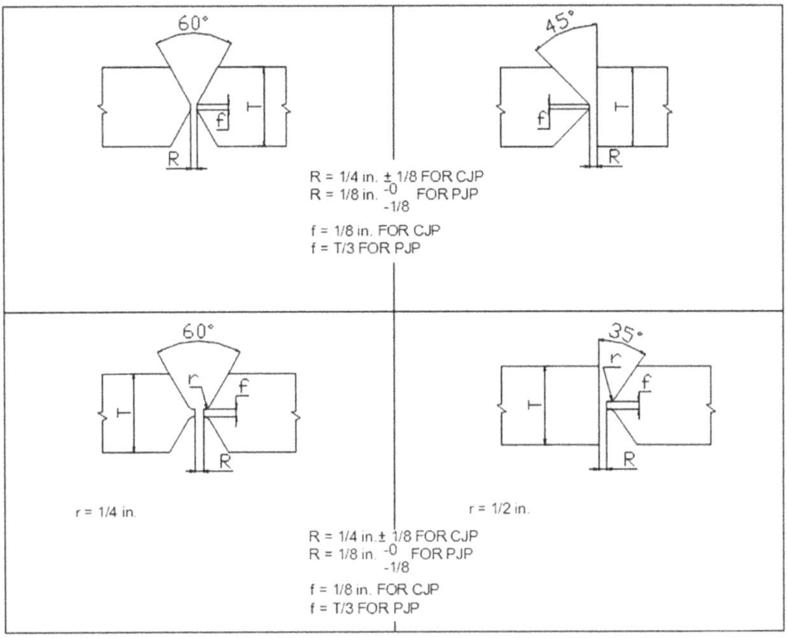

Figure 5.6 Suggested complete penetration and partial penetration groove designs.

minimum to ensure complete fusion. To avoid heat affected drawbacks, preheating before welding, must be adopted as it: (i) improves fusion of weld metal to obtain complete fusion; (ii) prevents cracking; (iii) reduces residual stresses; (iv) reduces distortion; (v) reduces hardness of the heat affected zone; (vi) reduces temperature gradients when welding thin to thick base metals and (vii) reduces temperature gradients when welding dissimilar base metals.

Peening: Peening is an option for controlling distortion or reducing cracking in the weldment. To ensure effective peening, each bead should get many moderate blows perpendicular to the weld surface instead of few heavy blows. A rounded diameter peening tool with a diameter of 1/2–3/4 in. (13–19 mm) or a ball peen hammer is considered ideal for the operation. The weld metal should not be allowed to cool below 1000°F (538°C), but elevated temperatures near red hot are preferred for any peening operation. A typical peening procedure involves using a reciprocating air hammer at 90 psi (600 kPa) on a weld as long as 3 in. (76 mm). The tip of the peening tool should be no wider than the weld bead and have a tip radius half the tip width. Travel speed for peening is recommended to be 30–40 in. (750–1000 mm) per minute.

Cooling: The rate of cooling and the final residual stress are closely related. Rapid cooling increases residual stress and vice versa. By burying the casting in sand, post heating the welded casting with a torch or a heater, and covering the casting with an insulating blanket, cooling can be decelerated, which in turn reduces residual stress levels.

Post weld heat treatment (PWHT) [5]: It is a process to improve the ductility and machinability of the weld, to dissolve the cementite formed during welding, to transform martensite to a less brittle phase structure and to relieve residual stresses. To avoid thermal stress cracking caused by temperature variations in the casting, the post weld heating and cooling rates when heat treating large or complex castings should not exceed 55°C per hour. In some cases, a slower cooling rate is preferable.

5.2.2.4 Welding issues related to steel structure

Steel structure welding requires a good level of control in order to achieve reliability in the finished product. The welding of thick and thin structural plates require different control strategy.

Thin steel plate material issues: It is widely acknowledged that thin plate deformation can never be completely eliminated. As a result, residual heat straightening must be done in a way that does not harm the plate structure or properties while also being as cost-effective as possible. These specific requirements will be met if the straightening process is carried out using induction heating [6]. Recent research has revealed that the steel structure deforms proportionally to the increase in hardness, but this has little or no effect on toughness. Induction heating, for example, is ideal for large open structures but it has some constraints in small tight spaces. In these cases, the gas heating process is more practical [7].

Thick steel plate material issues: Distortion is not an issue in thick sections, but maintaining acceptable properties in the heat affected zone (HAZ) is the most difficult. There is a relationship between the HAZ width and welding heat input, the greater the heat input, the wider the HAZ. Titanium can be added to develop the potential to control the growth of austenite grains in the HAZ to reduce cracking sensitivity and improve toughness [8]. Hydrogen-induced cracking is also a significant phenomenon in multi-pass welded structures. It could be reduced by using low hydrogen consumables with less than 2.4 ppm.

5.2.2.5 Gas welding

Oxyacetylene flame is probably the most widely used for gas welding because of its high flame temperature (3200°C). In the oxyacetylene process, the metal is heated by the hot flame of a gas-fed torch. In the *neutral flame*, equal amounts of oxygen and acetylene is used. It has a blue inner core with a temperature of 3200°C. In the *carburizing flame*, there is an excess amount of acetylene with a temperature of 3100°C. In the *oxidizing flame*, the presence of oxygen is more. It is much bluer in color with a temperature of 3300°C.

5.2.2.6 Important welding factors

Recently, the Bureau of Energy Efficiency (BEE) published the following remarks for the procurement of arc welding technologies for energy conservation:

- Welding equipment should have energy saving mode while not in operation.
- Use of inverter-based equipment is essential for saving energy.
- The target power factor of the usable welding machine must be 0.9 and above.

In addition, thrust must be given on skill development of welders so that new and better technologies may be utilized. Following factors must be ensured:

- The welder must be able to read and interpret technical parameters/documents and identify the materials and tools required.
- The welder must be able to complete tasks while keeping safety rules, accident prevention regulations and environmental protection requirements in mind.
- While performing jobs, the welder must be able to apply professional skills, knowledge and core skills.
- The welder must be able to check the job/assembly for functionality, as well as identify and correct errors in the job/assembly.
- The welder must be able to document the technical parameters of the task at hand.

These factors may appear as insignificant and sometimes omitted from the manual of good welding practice but have a significant impact on the performance factor of any MSE involved in welding and manufacturing.

5.2.3 Metal casting

Casting is the most economical method to produce complex shape components (i.e., automotive, machine tools, pipe fittings, textile machinery) that would be difficult to make by other methods. Cast iron and aluminum are most commonly processed metals through this route. These metals in molten state are poured into a mold having the cavity of the desired shape so that metal takes an appropriate form on its solidification. With appropriate science of metal casting bronze, brass, steel, magnesium, zinc, etc. have also been casted [9].

Majorities of foundries fall in micro to small enterprises. These small foundries are still using cupolas using low ash metallurgical (LAM) coke and there is a need to switch these foundries to the induction melting route, considering the environment [10] aspects. Many improvements in foundry practices to enhance casting quality and overall productivity are also needed. In this section, emphasis is given on casting of aluminum alloys, SG iron and Dokra casting in regard to improve foundry practices at MSMEs.

5.2.3.1 Aluminum casting

There is a need to understand that sand testing is an essential prerequisite to know American Foundry Society – Grain fineness number (AFS GFN), clay content, permeability, etc. for building a sound sand-mold. Fine grain sand of GFN 70–90 is suitable for better surface finish. The value of permeability must be between 25 and 30 for escape of gases generated in the mold after casting (during solidification). To ensure the permeability and improve the plasticity of the mold to prevent defects like hot tears in the casting [11], the mold should be moderately rammed. More details of conventional aluminum casting are provided in Annexure-IV. For complex shapes, it is desirable to work on water-soluble cores. Cores are used to create the internal shape of the castings. If the internal shape is critical and the required surface roughness is better than 5 μm, conventional sand cores should not be used. For example, the fuel housing system of a gas turbine engine made of aluminum alloy has various interconnected internal channels for delivering metered quantity fuel. Given the intricacy of its internal structure, a conventional resin sand core is not suitable as it generates gas during casting that creates unwanted gas holes inside casting as well as the internal surface roughness does not come below 5 microns even after painting. In such cases water-soluble cores (composed of sugar, water-soluble binders and filler materials like alumina, zircon, etc.), which are highly soluble in water, can be used. The core is prepared by preparing slurry of ingredients in distilled water and pouring the slurry into a metallic core box. Once the core is set and dried, it is withdrawn from the core box and calcined at 800°C for two hours depending on its thickness. The calcinations process makes the core hard and removes the moisture from the core. The calcined core is to be used for casting of aluminum metals. Once casting is completed, the casting is immersed in water for core removal. The removal rate of water-soluble cores can reach up to 600 g/h. The compressive strength of this core is also very good to sustain the metallostatic pressure of the molten metal.

5.2.3.2 SG iron casting

The average productivity of widely used SG iron casting is 60–70% due to rejection on the shop floor and at the customer side. In order to increase the yield and improve the mechanical and other properties of SG iron, following scientific measures may be implemented:

- **Use of simulation software:** An average foundry develops 20–30 new castings every year. Each casting requires at least 2–3 trials. The average cost of each trial would be about Rs. 25,000 including the pattern modification, molding, pouring and inspection. The total trial cost for a new casting would be around Rs. 50,000 to Rs. 75,000. The total trial cost for a foundry per year would be Rs. 10 lakhs to Rs. 15 lakhs (in case of two trials and 20 new components per year). Even if all the trial scraps are sold separately, considering the average difference in the price of a salable casting and ferrous scrap metals as Rs. 30/kg and average rejection, the economic loss caused by defective castings, is Rs. 1500 per ton of production. There are about 5000 foundries in India producing nine million tons of ferrous castings. Therefore, the total economic loss of all Indian foundries will be around Rs.12,000 to 18,250 million [12]. To reduce this economic loss, casting simulation may be utilized to reduce the shop floor trials. Average casting simulation software (single user) costs about 20–30 lakhs. Therefore, it will be very cost-effective to use casting simulation before developing new casting even if a simulation engineer/method engineer is appointed by the foundry. The small foundries may approach research institutions or jointly buy simulation software and must perform precast simulations to save lots of resources and time.
- **Proper riser and gating design:** There is a misconception that SG iron castings associated with large risers contribute to lower yields. Several attempts have been made to make riserless castings for some of the items in a foundry. It is worth mentioning that if the riser is piped properly, then it not only improves the average yield of the concerned foundry but it also decreases rejections like bending, swelling, etc.; otherwise, it will act as a part of casting, creating more problems [13]. To avoid confusion, an engineer should begin the simulation with no riser (in case of ductile iron (DI)) and if the simulation shows a defected product with no riser, then an appropriate riser should be introduced. If sound casting is indicated by the software but also indicates some defect, then the method engineer improves piping of the riser (i.e., increase riser size, check metallurgical parameters like carbon equivalent and other compositions and incorporate corrections, correct pouring temperature, checking modulus of the riser neck and in-gate and incorporate corrections) to remove all the defects. If

possible, for lightweight parts, stack molding may be introduced to enhance yield up to a great extent.

- **Inoculation:** The inoculation process creates a nucleation center for precipitating graphite into small flakes that evenly gets distributed throughout the matrix. By inoculation, the following improvement can be achieved:
  - Improved mechanical properties of gray or SG iron.
  - Control of graphite structure.
  - Reduction of iron carbide.
  - Reduction of casting section sensitivity.
  - Reducing undercooling.

There are mainly two types of inoculation: ladle (pot) and late (delayed) inoculation. With pot inoculation, the inoculant is added when the molten iron enters the pot or shortly thereafter. Delayed inoculation is treatment after leaving the pot, for example, when entering the mold (stream inoculation) or by using an insert in the mold (stream inoculation). The inoculum reaches its maximum effect shortly after treatment and declines rapidly over a period of 10–20 minutes. Therefore, it is desirable to inoculate as late as possible before watering. Pouring stream inoculation is being practiced at Council of Scientific and Industrial Research-Central Mechanical Engineering Research Institute (CSIR-CMERI) and it has been found that the counts of modularity increase significantly as compared to ladle inoculation [14].

5.2.3.3 Dokra casting

Dokra casting (also known as clay molded investment casting "CMIC") process is an ancient tradition of Asia, Africa and Pan-Pacific regions and is still followed in many regions of India, Bangladesh, Papua New Guinea and Benin of West Africa. This cost-effective casting process is easy to implement [15]. As this process is very common to various micro and small foundries, the process in brief and suggested solutions of problems related to Dokra casting are described in Annexure-IV.

5.3 SKILL ENHANCEMENT

The growth of a nation and strength of a country can be judged by the knowledge and skills acquired by its human resources. In the present scenario education is important but skill with knowledge is more important; therefore, skill enhancement programs play a key role in increasing productivity and reducing poverty. Skill is the ability to use the learned knowledge effectively in executing/performing a particular task to achieve the desired results. The skills required to perform general tasks are: time management, teamwork, self-motivation, etc. However, there are the domain-specific skills (i.e., welding, milling, casting), which are required for the successful execution of a specific task/certain jobs. To provide domain-specific skills, enhancing the productive capabilities through learning is emphasized. The main intention of the skill development program is to enable the individuals to acquire the capabilities to meet the changing demands and to encourage them to adopt these capabilities to increase their productivity by which they can earn a good amount to lead better livelihoods and also to grab the opportunities of economy and labor market. The types of skills required for employment can be divided into:

- Basic/foundation skills: Active learning, oral expression, reading comprehension, written expression, information and communication technology (ICT) literacy, active listening, etc. are the preliminary requirements for acquiring further skills.
- Technical skills: Acquiring of specialized skills, knowledge or know-how to perform specific tasks mainly in a professional environment is categorized as technical skills. Abilities to learn and adapt, solve problems, communicate ideas effectively, think critically and creatively to adapt themselves to different work environments as well as improving their opportunities for career-building play a key role as a crucial vehicle for social equity and sustainable development.
- Personal skills: Individual attributes relevant to work such as honesty, integrity, reliability, work ethic and judgment are considered as professional and personal skills. These skills play an important role in the overall growth of the individual employee and also in the sustainable development of the organization he or she works in.

Each country should have suitable infrastructure to provide both hard skills as well as soft skills to generate sufficient supply of manpower to be utilized in the industry, which in turn will help in the improvement of industrial economy, the professional network, better communication, time management and negotiation skills. Many of the MSME sectors are not given importance due to the reason that their low capital involvement and "skill gap" act as major hurdles. Skill gap is a gap between the current capabilities of an organization and skills that are required for the successful achievement of their planned goals in the coming future.

In the present situation, it is very difficult to get quality labor, the lack of which hampers the overall growth and prospects of the sector. Poor education during the initial level of life is the main reason for the lack of availability of quality labor. In addition, absence of vocational training is another reason. It is a proven fact that productivity cannot be increased without employee's development. Hence, the primary requirement of any organization is to provide continual training to its workforce.

Research institutions, having vast infrastructure and sound knowledge-base, can put efforts to uplift the MSME sector by interacting with many nearby MSMEs, understanding their needs and supporting them by providing technical know-how as well as training to solve their long-standing problems and enabling them to be a strong player in the present competitive and challenging market. The range of interventions includes identification, cluster institution partnership, outreach activities, common facility center (CFC) creation and technology infusion and capacity utilization. The major problems that the most of small enterprises face in terms of technology needs and other associated issues are:

- Poor quality consciousness.
- Lack of awareness about pollution abatement measures preferred by organized markets.
- Practicing the same age-old traditional method of production.
- Low or no upgradation with the current trends in technological development.
- Frequent occurrence of manufacturing defects and high rejection rates.
- Lack of testing raw materials and final products.

Intervention of research institutions in regard to technological infusion and skill development in some of these above clusters are discussed here briefly. To help clusters (units consisting of 100–1000 micro–small enterprises), often the need for developing special-purpose machines emerges. One such requirement came from a cluster of ferrous and non-ferrous metal part (1000 micro and small units, about 5000 manpower) manufacturers. Possible R&D infusion in anchor bolt manufacturing through the metal injection molding (MIM) route and upliftment of skill in regard to understanding of engineering drawing was required. Accordingly, CSIR-CMERI developed a special-purpose machine that reduces the process time of anchor bolt manufacturing by around 40%. The details of the machine are given in the next section. Similarly, the metal injection molding process as a near net shape manufacturing route has been introduced to the cluster by developing one of their high-volume production components, namely, copper nozzle [16]. The copper nozzles are commonly manufactured by conventional machining from hexagonal copper bars. Wastage of material and low production volume enhances the manufacturing cost of the nozzle. However, copper nozzles manufactured to the final shape using tiny copper powder as raw material in MIM can reduce manufacturing cost by 20–25% as estimated by the cluster through reduction in material wastage, less rejection and involvement of less manpower. The developed copper nozzle is shown in Figure 5.7.

Makhana cluster, Malda, West Bengal: Makhana (gorgon nut) pop is a vital nutrient-dense food made from water resources of low-land environments in India. At present, a good number of people are engaged with the activities of making makhana pop. During the session, all the family

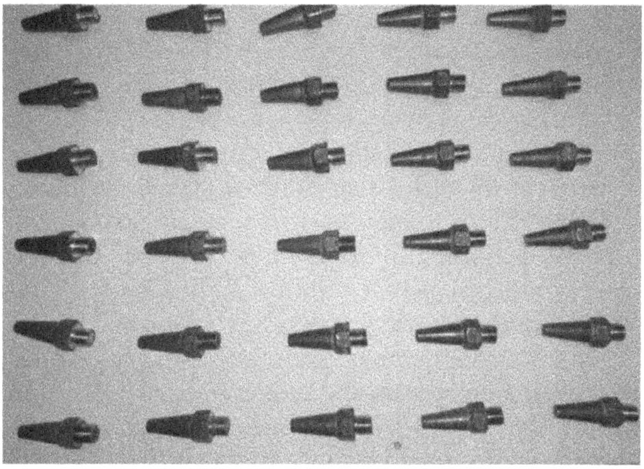

Figure 5.7 Copper nozzle developed through the MIM process.

members are involved with the traditional processing of makhana seed. Various processes performed after harvesting the makhana seed are: drying using sunlight and storage, sorting in different sizes, preheating, tempering, roasting, popping, polishing, grading and packaging. Among these processes, preheating, tempering and roasting are most drudgery and unhygienic because wood is used as the source of heating. Moreover, productivity is very poor as 4–5 manpower can produce an average of 1 kg of makhana pop per hour. The primary motivation to mechanize the process is to increase the production rate and maintain healthy and hygienic conditions. A completely new machine was developed, and subsequent to that development, the hands-on training on the developed machine was provided to MSME employees.

5.4 INTRODUCING NEW TECHNOLOGIES

To enhance productivity and bring product diversification, there is a need to percolate technological intervention in machines commonly used by micro and small industries. As the manufacturing sector is very diverse, technological intervention may be made according to the requirement. However, some of the new technologies such as special-purpose machines, micromachining and 3D printing may be very useful in the context of micro and small-scale manufacturing industries. Introducing special-purpose machines will definitely increase the productivity in case of high-volume production, micromachining will play an important role with the ever increasing miniaturization of the systems and 3D printing will increase the response time in regard to changing market demand.

5.4.1 Special-purpose machines

Generally conventional machines such as lathe, drilling machine, milling machine, hydraulic press, etc. are used in micro and small industries for component manufacturing. Since these are general purpose machines, productivity does not increase in the case of high production requirements for a particular type of component. In such circumstances, special-purpose machines (to perform specific operations to manufacture a specific component to increase productivity by 3–10 times [17]) are the best solution. The special-purpose machines are designed to operate round the clock and minimize "human errors and fatigue" in the repetitive work. Special-purpose machines may be of manual, semi-automatic or fully automatic type. It may be stand-alone or integrated type, depending on the requirement. Conventional machines sometimes can be converted to special-purpose machines with addition of special attachment or special fixture to attract micro and small industries because of their cost-effectiveness. Few examples of such special-purpose machines, made for micro/small enterprises, are given below:

5.4.1.1 Slitting machine for anchor bolt manufacturing

Anchor bolts are primarily employed to attach objects to the concrete [18]. One side of the anchor bolt is anticipated to be fixed in concrete while the other side is kept projected from the concrete for anchoring objects. Depending on the object type and load, anchor bolt ends particularly the fixed end in concrete are required to be designed [19]. It follows the standard ASTM F1554-18.

Various types of concrete anchors are used depending on the application such as acoustical wedge anchors, drop-in anchors, double expansion shield anchors, KapToggle hollow, lag shield expansion, machine screw, plastic toggle, Sammy screws, sleeve type, toggle wing hollow wall anchors, wedge anchors, hammer drive pin anchors, etc. In this chapter, a special-purpose machine is described with the aim to reduce the production cycle time of hammer drive pin anchor bolts toward increasing its production rate.

Hammer drive pin type anchor bolts (as shown in Figure 5.8(i)) is one of the simplest types, and it is employed for lighter objects. It consists of four components, namely, pin, nut, washer and bolt. One end of the bolt is threaded and the other end is grooved (folds) and slitted for a particular length. The slit width is normally kept as 1 mm. A through stepped hole (smaller diameter in the grooved side and a comparatively larger diameter on the other side so that it can allow the pin to enter) is present inside the anchor bolt. First a hole of slightly larger diameter than the anchor bolt is drilled on the concrete. Then, the debris inside the hole is removed. The anchor bolt along with the pin inside it is inserted into the hole. Now, a hammer is driven into the exposed head of the drive pin. As a result, it expands the anchor bolt base creating a grip inside the masonry material as shown in Figure 5.8(ii).

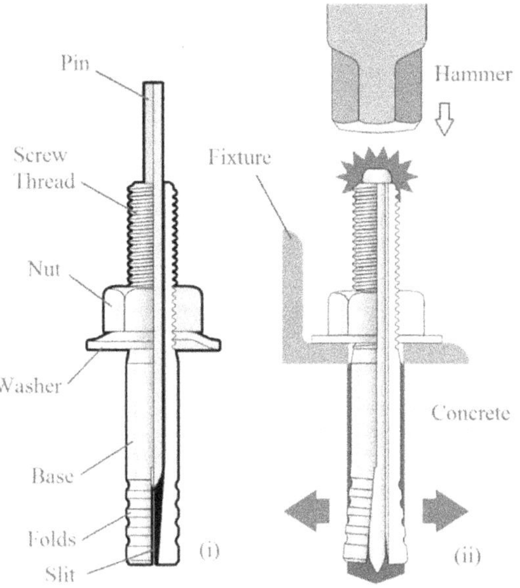

Figure 5.8 Architecture of a typical hammer drive pin type anchor bolt.

Conventional production cycle of the pin type anchor bolt (body) followed by micro and small industries comprises a number of sequential machining operations, namely, shearing (for the desired length), facing, grooving, drilling and finally slitting. Among these operations, stilling is found to consume more time 13 sec per piece and it is most dangerous as the operation is performed by pushing the bolt against a rotating cutting blade. In order to overcome these drawbacks, a semi-automatic multi-point slitting machine is designed and prototyped as shown in Figure 5.9.

The machine has two cutting blades for making slots simultaneously on two anchor bolts. A job-holding disk which accommodates eight anchor bolts rotates continuously. The cutting operations and loading/unloading the job are carried out simultaneously, thus making the machining process continuous. According to the design calculation, considering indexing speed 1 rpm, the slitting time per anchor bolt comes to 7.5 sec which is lower than the 13 sec required for conventional slitting operation. It is found that simultaneous slitting operations on both the anchor bolts are performed smoothly corresponding to a 1 hp motor with 1440 rpm.

5.4.1.2 Machine for manufacturing of surgical tools

A special-purpose machine, with necessary cutting tools and fixtures for machining of different geometric features of surgical tools is shown in Figure 5.10. Presently, different features of surgical tools are being machined

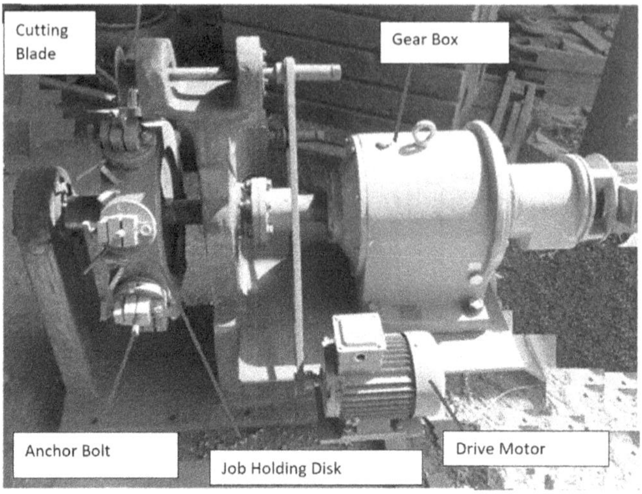

Figure 5.9 Prototype of a semi-automatic special-purposed slitting machine.

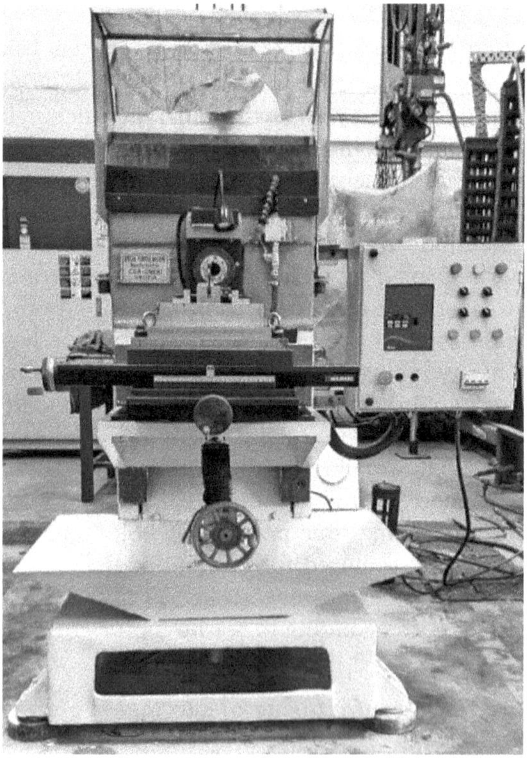

Figure 5.10 A special-purpose machine for machining different geometries of surgical tools.

manually which takes more time, and the component rejection rate is quite high due to lack of repeatability in the manual process. Initially, Spencer Wells straight artery forceps is identified as the first tool for its wide application and demand. Accordingly, all cutters and fixtures are designed and manufactured by CSIR-CMERI. Different features of the forceps like serration, lock profile and slots have been machined and demonstrated using the special-purpose machine. Though, the machine developed can be deployed for machining of geometric features of other similar surgical tools by altering the cutting tools and work-holding fixtures.

5.4.2 Micromachining

Micro manufacturing is commonly understood as the generation of high precision components with sizes ranging from tens of micrometers to a few millimeters utilizing different materials and processing techniques [20]. Automotive, aerospace, optics, electronics, biomedical, aviation, IT and other relevant industries are the major beneficiary of this rapidly evolving new technology. Between 2019 and 2025 global micro electromechanical system (MEMS) revenue alone among all microengineered components is expected to grow from the US $11.5 billion to the US $17.7 billion at a 7.4% compound annual growth rate (CAGR) [20]. Micromanufacturing processes can be broadly classified into five categories [21]:

- Subtractive processes (micromachining).
- Additive processes (surface coating, microcasting, microinjection molding, etc.).
- Deforming processes (microforming, hot embossing, micro/nano-imprinting, etc.).
- Joining processes (micromechanical assembly, laser welding, vacuum soldering, etc.).
- Hybrid processes (microlaser electro chemical machining (ECM), Lithographie, Galvanoformung, Abformung (LIGA), laser-assisted microforming, etc.).

The most commonly used process among the above five is the subtractive micromachining. The global micromachining market is expected to grow from US $2.4 billion in 2020 to US $3.3 billion by 2025 at a CAGR of 6.2%, driven mainly by the growing demand for microelectronics and microscale biomedical components [22]. During the last decade, the automobile sector was the most prominent end user of micromachined components; a typical application of which is a diesel injector [23]. Different micromachining techniques are also becoming useful for the diamond and jewelry industries. Synova SA manufacturer of laser micromachines, has established the world's largest diamond cutting and polishing center (Synova Micro-Machining Centre, India) in Surat (India) for providing service to different small diamond industries [24]. This contributes toward less weight loss, reduced cutting time, minimized damages to precious rough stones and overall increased yield to the diamond jewelry makers. Other than diamond, micromachining is becoming rapidly popular among titanium, platinum and gold jewelry makers for better productivity, precise design. Different micromachined parts are also becoming inevitable for surgical tools, automobiles, die and punch for electronics and horological applications, aerospace components, MEMS, optics and microfluidic applications. Developing/opening-up facilities and expertise required for micromachining will be useful for societal growth and development in the field of manufacturing, machine development, energy and allied areas. Figure 5.11 shows paper fuel cell

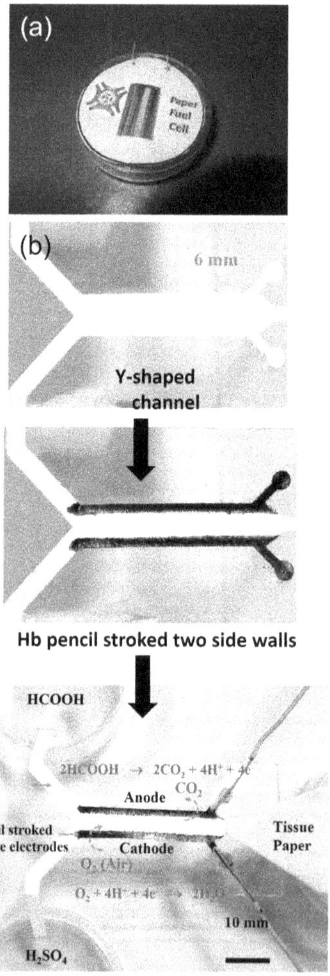

Figure 5.11 a) Paper fuel cell. b) Microfluidic channel manufactured by micromachining at CSIR-CMERI.

microfluidic paper channels developed for small-scale energy application. Paper channels used for development of these channels are generated using a universal CO_2 laser micromachine, whereas in Figure 5.12 a micropatterned SS stamp for hot embossing on glass is being shown. Stamps developed in this activity were used for transferring patterned features on photovoltaic glass substrates for increasing efficiency of solar cells.

Micromachining, a process of creating features in the order of micrometers (10^{-6} of a meter), demands unprecedented accuracy and high precision in machine tools. These microparts are used in a myriad of applications ranging from precise and sharp surgical tools used in healthcare to highly polished optical mirrors/reflectors used in the aerospace industry. The Multi-Fab (Figure 5.13) developed at CSIR-CMERI is fully indigenous in terms of its controller, graphical user interface (GUI) and all other hardware subsystems. CSIR-CMERI developed a desktop size micromachine capable of performing four operations and creating complex features/shapes in the dimension scale of 0.1–3 mm over a range of materials. The machine can be reconfigured for various machining operations as shown in Figure 5.13a.

CSIR-CMERI has developed two micromachines (Figure 5.13b) for small and micro scale industries and skill development initiatives. The first variant (LHS of Figure 5.13b) is capable of performing microdrilling, micromilling, microturning and microshaping operations in a single station. Being equipped with an indigenous controller and a GUI, the machine has become a perfect solution to numerous problems of small-scale jewelry, biomedical and optics industries. Many problems related to the generation

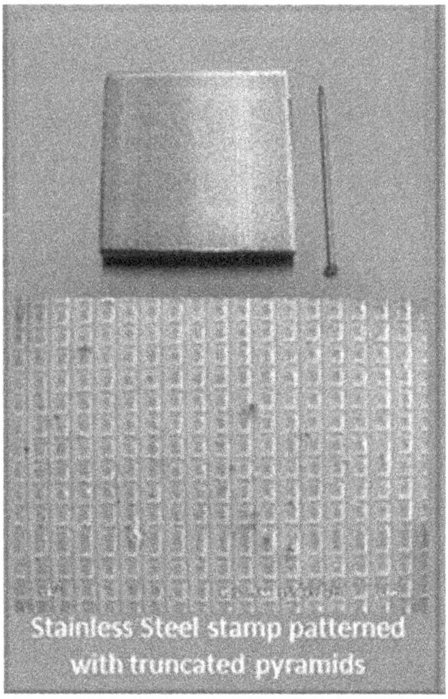

Figure 5.12 Micropatterned SS stamp for hot embossing on glass (energy application).

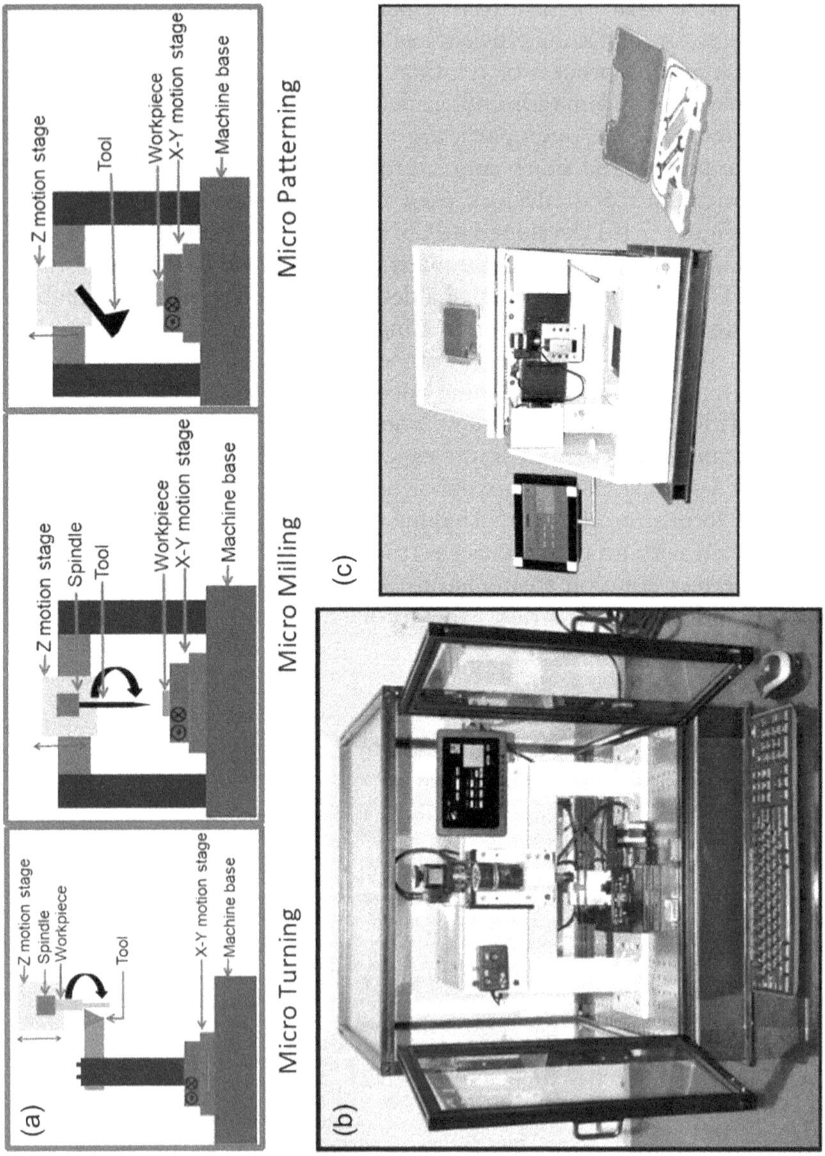

Figure 5.13 a) Schematic of Multi-Fab operations. b) Two variants of Multi-Fab developed at CMERI.

of microscale features with improved quality and repeatability of different micro and small-scale industries are being economically resolved by introducing the Multi-Fab machine. The second variant (RHS of Figure 5.13b), apart from having all features of the first variant, is capable of machining of microscale non-metallic features by using laser machining technique. These machines are also playing a crucial role in skill development related to CNC classes to educate engineering students. The rationale behind this is to provide the technology aid for future engineers and technicians to cultivate their skill through active learning, which is one of the major bottlenecks in most of engineering education institutions. One of the reasons would be non-affordability of the costly facilities and their regular maintenance.

5.4.3 3D printing

The terminology for 3D printing is very common and often it is referred to as additive manufacturing process. There are a number of feasible concepts related to additively depositing material to build a part, but ASTM Committee F42 has categorized additive manufacturing processes into seven subgroups, i.e., binder jetting (BJ), directed energy deposition, material extrusion, material jetting, powder bed fusion (metals: DMLS, SLM; polymers: SLS), sheet lamination and vat photo-polymerization.

5.4.3.1 3D printing process

Following five core steps remain consistent across all 3D printing processes:

Producing a 3D file: The user designs or "models" the desired 3D object using computer-aided design (CAD) tools. There are primarily three types of modeling techniques – solid modeling, free form surface modeling and digital sculpting. For small-scale industries, solid modeling is relatively cost-effective due to its widespread usage, powerful features and versatility across platforms. To print 3D parts, the first step is to create a digital model using computer-aided design (CAD) software. Reverse modeling can also be used to create CAD models by scanning actual parts. When planning for 3D printing, several design constraints must be considered. These generally concentrate on feature geometry constraints, support material requirements and escape hole requirements. To 3D print a part, a CAD model must be converted into a format that a 3D printer can understand. This is accomplished by first converting the CAD model into a STereoLithography (STL) file, also known as a Standard Triangle Language file. Two other formats OBJ and 3DP are also acceptable 3D printing file formats, but they are less popular. STL describes an object's surface areas using triangles (polygons), simplifying the complex CAD model. After creating an STL file, it is uploaded into a program, which slices the design into the layers which will be used to construct the part. The slicing process converts the

3D model design into horizontal cross-sectional layers and allows the user to determine a toolpath, speed, orientation, etc.

The slicer program transforms the STL file into G-code. G-code is a numerical control programming language used in computer-aided manufacturing (CAM) to control automated machines such as CNC machines and 3D printers. The slicer program also allows the 3D printer controller to describe the build parameters of the 3D printer by identifying the support location, layer height and part orientation. Even though some universal slicer programs exist, such as Netfabb, Simplify3D and Slic3r, slicer programs are often proprietary to every brand of 3D printer.

Printing: Despite the aid of computer systems, the first few steps are semi-automated which necessitate significant manual control, interaction, and decision-making. After such steps, the process moves on to the computer-controlled building phase. All 3D printing machines will deposit layers with a height adjustable platform or deposition head, deposition mechanisms and layer formation. Some machines combine material deposition and layer formation at the same time, while others separate them. As long as no errors are detected during the build, 3D printing machines will keep layering until the job is finished [25].

Material removal/cleanup: The part manufactured in additive manufacturing (AM) may preferably be ready for use directly. However, it is not always true, more often produced parts will require post-processing before use. The manufactured part is first separated from the build platform and then excess build material must be removed. Sometimes removal may require a wire electrical discharge machining (EDM) machine, band saw and/or milling equipment. Part removal requires a certain level of operator skill because mishandling of parts and poor technique can result in part damage. Cleanup requirements vary depending on the 3D printed part. The cleanup stage is the first stage of post-processing. To achieve final properties, post-processing may involve chemical treatment or heat treatment of the part. Because different 3D printers produce varying degrees of accuracy, machining to final dimensions may be required. Some processes generate comparatively delicate components, which may necessitate the use of intrusion and/or surface coatings to strengthen the finished product. The use of power tools, CNC milling and additional equipment, such as polishing tubs or drying and baking ovens, can benefit some of the post-processing tasks [25].

5.4.3.2 Selection of 3D printing methods

This section focuses on the use of additive manufacturing to generate final parts for micro and small businesses and the obvious choice will be among

BJ, DMLS, SLS and SLM to achieve higher strength and functionality in printed parts.

5.4.3.3 Business opportunities and future directions

To recover from the pandemic situation and ensure the long-term viability of MSMEs, characteristics of business models based on longevity, renewability, reuse, repair, upgrade, refurbishment, capacity sharing and dematerialization must be identified. MSMEs frequently use the Internet (Web) to gather product ideas and then modify product shape/features based on their accessible manufacturing facilities. To replace product development and its distribution business model, "additive manufacturing and digital interface" must be added. The key stages of the new business model innovation process are design improvement or reconfiguration of existing products at the local level, as AM allows digital designs to be transformed into physical products anywhere in the world. Using web tools (digital interface) to add features related to "local manufacturing" and "easily available materials" help to spread product ideas and component designs and leads to new models of entrepreneurship for MSMEs. This type of digital entrepreneurship is the way of the future for MSMEs.

Digital entrepreneurship has the potential to generate decentralized and sustainable jobs that are not vulnerable to pandemic/lockdown/social unrest. This form of employment is not prone to off-shoring since it is based on a distributed network, where cost of "internet facilities including digital interface" is a fraction of the total costs. The creating, capturing value and delivering products through change in one or many components in the existing business model will assist in setting up virtual enterprises incorporating "digital marketing", "technology sharing" and "material selection" characteristics [26]. This kind of business opportunities may require leasing the AM equipment like document printers as of current scenario, which ultimately reduce "equipment cost". Some additional features like post-processing of products after production and automating delivery systems may be required.

5.5 IMPLEMENTATION OF SMART MANUFACTURING

In this section, an overview of smart manufacturing and Industry 4.0 are discussed. These topics have been described considering benefits, challenges and possible impact on the micro and small enterprise (MSE) sector. The participation of MSE sectors in automobile parts, machine components, metallic and electronics items, medical equipment, microelectro components, etc. [27] is continuously increasing. The micro and small enterprises are getting proactive in improving their business operations by adopting a concept of Industry 4.0 [28], which aims to attain the effective utilizations of ICT in the manufacturing environment. It is also focused to bring global transformation in manufacturing and upgradation so that MSEs will grow potentially with low investment along with more operational flexibility and less location-wise mobility. This brings basically the concept of Internet of things (IoT) applications with servitization in the manufacturing environment [29]. "The Industry 4.0 is a collective term for technologies and concepts of value chain organization. Within the modular structured smart factories of Industry 4.0, Cyber-Physical System (CPS) monitors physical processes, creates a virtual copy of the physical world, and makes decentralized decisions. Over the IoT, CPSs communicate and cooperate with each other and humans in real-time. Via the Internet of Service (IOS), both internal and cross-organizational services are offered and utilized by participants of the value chain [30]". This adds smartness to MSEs by providing a robust sectoral digital platform to strengthen its mandate for the benefit of enterprises and boosting their networks through digital communications sources. This also helps in developing the concept, design analysis, real-time process control, observation and feedback from the customers directly through this digital/smart manufacturing. Therefore, MSEs can improve their product quality, efficiency by reducing operating costs to deliver successful products and grow in a faster manner in the market.

5.5.1 Description and implementation of Industry 4.0 in smart manufacturing

Typically, the Industry 4.0 concept covers smart product design, smart machining processing, smart monitoring systems, smart control systems, smart scheduling and its manufacturing/industrial applications. To implement Industry 4.0, the manufacturing sector focuses on developing products from a new design to suitable applications, establishing a model for the design of manufacturing systems to prove "the suitability of cyber-physical system (CPS)" and "smart product design concept" [31]. Predictive maintenance and diagnosis of the machine health using CPS features are also added to Industry 4.0 concept. Machine Tool 4.0 features are also introduced in machining sites for attempting the next generation of machine tool systems. For attempting efficient decision-based energy systems, Energy Management 4.0 features will also be added to monitor and supply the required power to the manufacturing systems in a self-optimized manner [32]. A modified framework for smart manufacturing systems using the CPS [33] is shown in Figure 5.14. Another CPS feature in Industry 4.0 is the deployment of sensors and actuators for precise control, data collection, big data analysis and self-driven decision-making systems. The steps for Industry 4.0 to achieve a smart manufacturing environment are also shown in Figure 5.14.

	Smart Product Design	Smart Machining Process	Smart Monitoring System	Smart Control System	Smart Scheduling for Applications
Big Data Driven Decision	Data driven design	Data driven machining	Data driven (Real-time) monitoring	Data driven (Real-time) control	Data driven (Real-time) Scheduling
Big Data Analysis	Data driven analysis	Machine data analysis	Monitoring data analysis	Control data analysis	Scheduling data analysis
Data Collection	Design Data Collection	Machine Data Collection	Monitoring Data Collection	Control data Collection	Scheduling data Collection
Sensor & Actuators Deployment	Design oriented sensor deployment	Machine Oriented Sensor & actuator deployment	Sensor deployment for monitoring	Control Oriented Sensor deployment	Scheduling data Collection

Figure 5.14 Steps to achieve smart manufacturing environments.

For developing a smart product design in the smart manufacturing environment, the CPS provides the solution to enable smart machine tool systems to produce physical products which connect all the physical and virtual systems by creating a network system for communication and interaction of the intelligent devices with each other. This also provides the solution for smart production and scheduling systems toward manufacturing/industrial applications where the smart devices are digitally connected by the end-to-end feature of the ICT system [32]. The radio frequency identification device (RFID) tags, Zigbee and Wi-Fi modules are attached to key element components (like bearings, spindles and cutting tools, etc.) for connecting physical objects using unique identification address protocols. During the operation of the machine tool system, a variety of sensors and actuators such as dynamometers, temperature sensors, vibrations sensors, cameras and its support acquisition devices are integrated with the systems to monitor real-time machine performance. The machining process data are collected by attached key elements. The different data communication technologies such as RS-232, Ethernet, Bluetooth, 3G/4G network, etc. are exploited for transmitting the real-time data. For gathering all the data, all key components are to be defined so that their physical characteristics and real-time status can be simultaneously identified. The communication protocols are standardized so that communications are carried out properly where MTConnect standards are used for identification of manufacturing equipment because these communication standards are easily available. Therefore, a plug-and-play environment can be used in the manufacturing environment which reduces the cost of data integration [34]. MTConnect can interpret collected data from different devices into a common format (like XML, etc.) which is used by most software applications. An ISO-10303 file is also created which is known as a STEP format. Using said standard protocols, the communication service (through the internet service provider) sends the communication to the key components and collects real-time data for a particular application.

Smart visibility consists of two parts, i.e., controllability of devices and monitoring of data which can be developed using a user interface (UI) application. The most advantages of such kinds of applications are in collecting real-time data with the help of communication services. All key components of smart machine tools can be remotely controlled and monitor the data from a PC or mobile devices, etc. The statistical reports can be generated directly for business management systems like enterprise resource planning (ERP), etc. to make an effective decision-making system for predictive maintenance and diagnosis of the machine health or any failure, etc. All statistical data are stored in the cloud and different artificial intelligence algorithms can be applied for the prediction of the demand of the market. Virtual and augmented reality can help during the visualization of exact machining processes. Using such technologies, real-time manufacturing data can be collected during machining processes to enable instinctive and efficient interactions and collaboration between smart machine tools and users.

5.5.2 Key elements/components of smart manufacturing

Smart manufacturing must ensure that the following seven essential critical technology elements are present as building blocks toward developing a smart manufacturing environment [35].

Smart devices: Smart devices bridge "intelligent functionality" with "existing industrial control systems" and provide an automation solution. An intelligent functionality of smart devices offers suitable communication, control functions and computations within networking systems using smart hubs/gateways.

Smart user interfaces (UIs): A smart user interface (UI) provides a user-friendly interface to connect human with machines and facilitates remote monitoring and control of smart devices The device-to-device, device-to-equipment and equipment-to-equipment connectivity can also be established using smart UIs where information technology (IT)/operation technology (OT) interfaces between the two systems via the industrial IoT. Such an interface plays a vital role in modern, micro and small industries. This improves the production rate in the manufacturing environment, automated delivery and diagnostics, etc.

Edge computing devices: The edge computing devices provide intelligence and control at each hierarchical level of the manufacturing system which can be computed through sensor integration within the edge network and sends information immediately to the smart interface device. Also, it provides information to centralized IT data management systems and industrial control system software so that the decision can be made at the right time at the right machine location for increasing productivity and reducing downtime. This helps in the improvement of the quality of the product during product handling devices in a different industry.

Software platforms and apps: The software platforms and apps provide intelligent functionality within the manufacturing system using smart UIs and edge computing devices. These consist of bundled with commercial-off-the-shelf smart devices and smart interfaces for machine tools. This also offers retrofit intelligent functionality which is freely available in mobile apps and desktop computers. Therefore, micro and small enterprises and start-ups can utilize those software.

Data management systems (DMSs): DMS offers the collection of data and its analysis for easily accessible relevancy which helps manufacturers boost the efficiency and reduce costs of the system. This also provides intelligent filters that require it across the MSEs.

Big data analytics: Big data analytics gives solutions toward analyzing the data using advanced analytical techniques (statistics tools, artificial intelligence and machine learning method, condition-based maintenance, prognostics, etc.) which helps in the prediction of the health of any machine or any failure that was previously unpredictable or unnoticeable. This will be helpful for preventive maintenance of the machine, life expectancy and reusability of machine tools in MSEs.

Safety and security: Safety and security are the most prominent functions for protection of any manufacturing system from the point of view of operator safety especially smart manufacturing where human–machine interactions and cyber security vulnerabilities in network security are linked with integration of IT/OT systems. This is another area of R&D for threat vulnerability in industrial IoT infrastructure which is to be configured properly to protect the smart manufacturing systems.

CSIR-CMERI is working on a project named “SMART Foundry”, to develop a complete advanced foundry for the casting of small aluminum components of up to 2 kg. The overall system foot print will fit inside a 12 ft × 12 ft room. More details of this project are provided in Annexure-IV.

5.5.3 Benefits and challenges of smart manufacturing

The number of micro–small enterprises is increasing because these units require less capital outlay but provide more employment and help in the development of economic status of the country. This is very useful for remote areas where the people have yet to be trained to meet the challenge of sophisticated technology [36]. To help small enterprises, there is a growing need for smart and digital technologies, to develop sophisticated but cost-effective, resource (energy, material)-efficient and environment-friendly products. Such technologies will increase the interest of youngsters in getting into manufacturing jobs and provide a number of benefits such as "increased productivity", "improved operations", "better/faster decision-making", "optimum utilization of resources", "efficient real-time tracking", "greater flexibility in meeting high-level last-minute changes", "detailed end-to-end product transparency in real-time", etc. By using this concept of smart manufacturing, most companies will realize a return of investment (ROI) on their investments within a short time [37] and will also help develop the different organizational structures of the MSEs to move in a faster manner with supply chain management to achieve competitiveness in the market.

In the MSEs sector, smart manufacturing has a lot of benefits but there are challenges of "establishing very good interaction among academic, R&D and industries", "maintenance of high-cost manufacturing infrastructure", "skilled workforce", etc. Various schemes like the "Digital MSME" Scheme for the promotion of ICT in the MSE sector have been launched by the Ministry of MSME, India, and a special promotion "Make in India" [38] has been started. This provides more employment, reduces regional imbalances, creates the industrialization evaluation in rural and underdeveloped areas and paves the path of more equitable distribution for increasing the income and wealth. Thus, growth in the MSEs can directly build the way to better equity and inclusion in the economy by implementing smart manufacturing.

5.6 MANUFACTURING ETHICS

Manufacturing ethics ensure that production activities will neither harm the user nor the societal stake holders. Production activities aim for the well-being of all involved and take care of the 5 M (man, machine, materials, money and moral). In short, ethics builds a sense of right and wrong in the organizations with a vision of a sustainable future without harming society or environment.

5.6.1 Importance of ethics

Everyone wants businesses to be fair, clean and beneficial to the society and the business environment. To ensure this, manufacturing houses need to abide by the rule of law, engage themselves in fair practices and competition among themselves, which will benefit the end user with a larger benefit to the system, society, similar organization and its stakeholders. Every working professional desires to do work for an organization that is fair and ethical in its practices with transparency. An organization driven by moral values is appreciated in the society. Institutions with good corporate governance and social responsibility initiatives are well respected in every atmosphere. When all management and working class with all directly or indirectly associated with industry come together in a common platform to align themselves for achieving the sustainable common goals, it boosts the morale of everyone associated. Improving the decision-making process by everyone's involvement with trust to each other and support plays a vital role. Decisions are driven by values.

Today, faster changes in technologies are affecting the safeguarding of our regulations. As an example, by the time law comes up with a regulation, newer technology with latest threats replacing the earlier one emerges. In this situation our ethical activities only will safeguard the society. Ethical manufacturing is an approach which mainly focuses on developing high quality of product and services. Ethical production helps to develop product with efficiency, safety and considering the health of the employees. There are certain other factors like ethical and legal factors, which when taken into account will help to reduce the use of energy by increasing energy efficiency and exploring technologies to find innovative manufacturing processes. The waste can be reduced by taking innovative initiatives in the manufacturing process to improve ethical practices. It helps to develop brand image by developing high quality of product and services by considering all legal and ethical business practices. The ultimate aim of ethical business practices is to develop high quality of product and services by considering the environmental impact of the manufacturing process. It enables developing a secure workplace environment by making employees ethically and legally responsible to ensure that the employees are not subjected to harassment or any other illegal treatment at the workplace. The organization should be safe for all employees by treating them fair and equal. The effective manufacturing process has clear expectations, fair pay, compliance audits, active support and zero tolerance. There should be careful planning for the development of manufacturing processes including appropriate packaging processes, use of eco-friendly material and sustainable business practices.

5.7 SAFETY

In the earlier heading, more emphasis was given on economic revival through start-up/small–micro industries. With an increasing number of MSMEs, there is a need to consider occupational safety and health (OSH). It appears that due to financial pressure, issues related to occupational safety and health in micro–small industries are much higher than in medium–large industries. There is a need for implementation of safety practices to achieve economic and social development [39, 40]. Priority of safety versus productivity at the workplace should be conveyed and clarified to the workers periodically. In small enterprises, communication lines are very strong, short and personal and it is very easy to implement simple solutions at short notice. This brings owners and managers/supervisors closure and offers the employees a true sense of social relationship and often a great range of autonomy. Some important guidelines on safety are:

- As it is well known that none of the small industries have the capacity to run an occupational health service center on their own, but they can comfortably run few of them by forming a group of small industries and funding the expenditures fractionally, this not only eases the financial load on each industry but also forms a bonding among many different industries.
- As all small industries may not be financially strong enough to fund a full-fledged medical facility, they can contribute some amount toward the treatment of their employees and their dependents by joining hands with nearby health centers including accidental and emerging services.
- In another way, a general practitioner can be hired for providing treatment services in his/her clinic and he/she can provide a visiting occupational health nurse periodically for offering education and treatment/training at the work place.
- As a first step, a center to provide training for the first-aiders among the workers in nearby small industries must be developed to handle minor situations like injuries etc. before the patients are shifted to the hospitals.
- A safety consultant can be hired to provide training on the health and safety of the employees which will help in reducing the number of accidental cases by following the safety guidelines at the workplace.

5.7.1 Safety measures at the workplace

Some of the basic safety precautionary measures to be taken at the workplace of micro and small enterprises related to manufacturing are as follows:

5.7.1.1 General safety

Industries must provide suitable safety equipment and uniforms for the employees. A safety committee consisting of members from both management and shop floor members must conduct safety meetings on a regular basis to assess the safety situation as well as to make action plans to avoid any possible mishaps to both the employees and the equipment. Similarly, employees must be provided with a suitable set of tools to carry out day-to-day activities; in addition, it is also necessary to display the safety instructions for the employees at appropriate places in the shop floor with meaningful messages and pictures about safety precautions and some of them are mentioned below:

- A first aid box with basic medicines is to be kept at a suitable place (easily approachable by everyone).
- The place of the first aid box should be properly earmarked at several places to avoid delay in finding it when needed.
- Medicines in the first aid box must be periodically checked and replaced to avoid shortage and use of expired medicines.
- Posters with proper pictures with explanation in local language must be displayed at various places about DO'S and DON'T'S in case of any accidents.
- Selected few workers should be trained on first aid procedures so that they can assist the injured person till he/she is shifted to a hospital.
- Supervisors and managers should be trained to handle the situation (in case of any mishaps) to avoid crowd gathering and unwanted incidents.
- Contact numbers of nearby hospitals/doctors/ambulances/police stations and fire stations should be displayed properly for easy access at the time of requirement.
- Some volunteers among the workers should be nominated to take care and accompany the patient during shifting from the workplace to hospital/home.
- Warning signs should be provided near the areas of high voltage, fire or any dangerous environment.

5.7.1.2 *Machine shop safety*

Machine shops or machines in a micro/small enterprise are generally placed haphazardly with temporary or loose electrical connections. Often the operators are untrained and unqualified making the situation vulnerable to accidents. The following safety measures are mandatory for a machine shop:

- Chips and metal scraps are to be removed on a regular basis to maintain a clean area.
- Posters with safety instructions are to be placed at appropriate places to remind the operators.
- Concept of "arm swing" space must be implemented firmly to reduce the occupational hazards to another worker working on a neighboring machine.
- Sufficient light should be provided at the workplace.
- Basic safety equipment like goggles, hand gloves, aprons and safety shoes should be provided for the operators.
- Principles of 5S: Follow the path of "5S" – sort, set in order, shine, standardize and sustain.

5.7.1.3 Welding shop safety

Welding involves fire and gases; therefore, possibilities of danger and safety precautions, as mentioned in ANSI Z49, must be known to welders. Important safety precautionary measures are to be strictly followed to avoid the chances of accidents. It is necessary to ensure (1) the "proper civil and electrical installation" and "good working condition" of welding equipment and (2) availability of "eye protection glasses" and "protective clothing suitable for the welder".

It is essential to keep the workplace clean and free from flammable/volatile/explosive materials. Ventilation must be mandatorily practiced near the place of welding of lead, cadmium, chromium, manganese, brass, bronze, zinc or galvanized steel so that the air through the workspace caused by an electrical device is efficiently circulated with the outside environment. The entire compressed gas cylinder, whether completely filled/partially filled/almost empty, must be handled with extreme care. When utilizing a scaffold/ladder to complete the welding above the ground level, make sure that the work surface is solid and properly secured. If possible, use a safety belt or lifeline. When welding in a damp or wet area, wear rubber boots and stand on a dry and insulated platform. Do not use the cables which are having cracks or bare spots in their insulation. Do not allow flame or sparks to hit hoses, regulators or cylinders. Some of the safety rules to be followed strictly during welding operation are given below:

Safety measures in arc welding [40]:

- Strictly avoid looking at the welding arc without wearing the proper eye protection.
- Inhaling of the fume plume during the arc welding process must be avoided.
- Welding in a confined space without taking special precautions is an open invitation to the hazard and hence it is to be avoided.
- Welding on containers that are filled with combustibles is to be avoided and if very unavoidable then it must be handled by taking all suitable special precautions.
- Sealed containers or compartments must be welded after providing proper air vents to evacuate the gases and fumes generated during welding and also follow all suitable safety precautions.
- Welding electrodes must be properly hung onto their suitable brackets when not in use and never allow the electrode to touch any compressed gas cylinder nearby.
- Used welding electrode stubs are hazardous waste and must be discarded following all rules.

Safety precautions for oxyacetylene welding and cutting [40]:

1. Always use soap solution to detect leaks in tight joints during inspection and avoid using gas flame.
2. The work area must be kept clean and free from items/materials that cause hazards as during flame cutting operation the sparks can travel 30 to 40 ft (10 to 15 m).
3. Always make sure that appropriate and purpose-intended torches are used while using oxygen and acetylene or other fuel gases.
4. Acetylene must never be used at a pressure in excess of 15 psi (103.4 K Pa), as higher pressure can cause an explosion.
5. Oil and grease in contact with oxygen may cause spontaneous combustion; hence, always avoid using oil, grease or any material on any apparatus or threaded fittings in the oxyacetylene or oxy fuel system.
6. Always make it a practice to follow the cracking (opening the valve of the cylinder slightly, then closing) procedure while assembling apparatus, operating gas cylinder valves before attaching regulators. This cleans the accumulated foreign material by blowing. Always make sure that all threaded fittings are clean and tight.
7. Always use this correct sequence and technique for lighting a torch:
   a. Acetylene cylinder valves must be opened in the first step.
   b. Then, open and turn the acetylene torch valve by 1/4 turn.
   c. Adjust the working pressure by using the adjusting valve handle after screwing the acetylene regulator.
   d. Acetylene torch valves must be turned off to purge the acetylene line properly.
   e. Then, the valve of the oxygen cylinder can be opened slowly.
   f. Then, open and turn the oxygen torch valve by 1/4 turn.
   g. Adjust the oxygen regulator screw to the desired working pressure.
   h. Then, turn off the oxygen torch valve.
   i. Now open the acetylene torch valve by 1/4 turn and light by using a friction type lighter.
   j. After ensuring proper settings, open the oxygen torch valve by 1/4 turn.
   k. Now adjust the flow rate of both acetylene and oxygen properly to get a neutral flame.
8. Always use this correct sequence and technique for shutting off a torch:
   a. First close the valve of the acetylene torch and then close the valve of the oxygen torch.
   b. Similarly, close the valve of the acetylene cylinder first followed by the oxygen cylinder valve.
   c. Release the pressure in the regulator and hose by opening both the torch valves of acetylene and oxygen.

d. Continue backing off of the regulator adjusting valve handle until no spring tension is felt.
e. Finally close both the torch valves.

5.7.1.4 Foundry shop safety

Most of the foundry works require handling high temperature (~1000°C) molten metals and are dealt by low paid foundry workers. The setting up of molds requires physical activities such as standing, squatting, sitting, etc., which increases the chances of burn injury. Keeping in mind the hazardous environment, the following safety measures must be adhered by the foundry industry:

- Adequate training/awareness must be given about safety.
- Appropriate mechanized chargers/trolleys to assist foundry activities.
- Designated places to keep raw material/coal/scrap, etc.
- Ready firefighting equipment at designated places.
- It is wiser to have a pile of dry sand and a shovel ready to put out the fire or to control metal spills.
- Handling hot tasks during cooler times of the day and maintenance activities in the cooler seasons to avoid chances of any mishaps.
- Protective footwear and gloves, spats, protective clothing for exposed skin such as arms and legs.
- Skimmers and other melting tools must be preheated before use.
- Wear respiratory protection gadgets while melting copper-base alloys (brass, bronze).

5.7.1.5 Electrical safety

Almost all the equipment in MSMEs are powered by electricity. However, negligence in regard to electricity causes fatal safety hazards. Furthermore, most of the time it has been observed that the short circuits are caused by wear and tear and become a major source of accidents in any industry. Therefore, electrical equipment and instruments must be regularly serviced to avoid accidents. Following safety measures are required to be taken in regard to electricity-related hazards:

- Utmost care must be taken in storing of flammable, combustible, toxic and other hazardous materials and all the designated areas must be equipped with appropriate firefighting equipment. Sufficient number of employees must be properly trained on how to use those firefighting devices.
- People should be made aware of the place of main switches by suitable indication so that power supply can be stopped immediately in case of any short circuit or fire mishaps.

- Avoid allowing untrained/non-licensed electricians to work on high power electrical equipment/apparatus unless they are under the supervision of qualified or trained electricians.

5.7.1.6 *Material handling safety*

Improper handling of materials by an untrained employee can cause many health hazards like acute and chronic injuries like slip disc, musculoskeletal disorders (MSDs) and other types of injuries (person performing work above shoulder height, below knees, at full reach distance, etc.). Handling of materials in any unplanned way (i.e., without the use of proper tools and equipment, handling special materials, liquids, chemicals, etc. without appropriate care) also can create major health hazards. Often wire ropes are used to clamp and carry the load. It is necessary to examine the wires before and after usage to avoid any damage caused by worn wires, broken wires, loose fasteners (nuts/bolts). Further load balancing (NO tilt, speed within limits, controlled friction, etc.) must be ensured as a necessary safety measure [41].

5.8 SUMMARY

The effective implementation of manufacturing technologies will play a very important role in increasing the productivity of all manufacturing industries. Majority of R&D institutes emphasize on the development and application of advanced/innovative technical interventions (i.e., additive manufacturing, IoT-based manufacturing) required by MSMEs and can provide economical solutions to micro to small enterprises. This book chapter highlights the standard operating procedures to be followed in different manufacturing processes to avoid the rejections in components. The common mistakes often made by MSME personnel in machining, casting and welding are elaborated and its remedies are discussed in detail. Also, the new trends in manufacturing such as special-purpose machines, micromachining and 3D printing, which are practiced globally, are introduced in this book chapter. The chapter covers the importance of skill development and safety aspects in MSMEs to revolutionize the productivity of small clusters and bring them to new horizons. Salient features of this chapter include:

- Mistakes in machining occur due to improper selection of cutting tools and cutting parameters, which leads to underproduction, underutilization of machine and/or cutting tools, premature failure of tools and/or machine parts.
- Defects in welding like porous weld, undercutting, distortions spatter, etc. occur due to too long/short arc length, too high welding current,

arc blow, etc. Awareness regarding appropriate process parameter selection will increase the productivity of weld products.
- Sand casting industries require sand testing, such as AFS GFN, clay content permeability, etc., prior to molding. Proper gating must be designed to allow the mold to fill rapidly with negligible turbulence. If possible, follow simulation of the casting process to ensure proper filling of the molds.
- There is a need to invest in skill development programs so that skilled manpower is available for industrial growth. This will increase the spread of technological interventions in majority of the manufacturers across the country. Some of the new technologies such as special-purpose machines, 3D printing, micromachining, Industry 4.0 integrated "advanced manufacturing technologies" and concept of servitization may be learnt via skill development programs.

BIBLIOGRAPHY

1. J. Norrish. *Advanced Welding Processes.* Woodhead Publishing, Elsevier, Cambridge, England 2006.
2. A.S. Whyte. The welding of cast iron. *New Zealand Engineering*, 3:176, 1948.
3. D.K. Dwivedi. *Design of Welded Joints: Weld Failure Modes, Welding Symbols: Type of Welds, Joints, Welding Position.* Springer, Singapore, 2022.
4. Y.M. Zhang, and S.B. Zhang. Double-sided arc welding increases weld joint penetration. *Welding Journal-Including Welding Research Supplement*, 77(6):57–62, 1998.
5. B.K. Srivastava, S.P. Tewari, and J. Prakash. A review on effect of preheating and/or post weld heat treatment (PWHT) on mechanical behavior of ferrous metals. *International Journal of Engineering Science and Technology*, 2(4):625–631, 2010.
6. N.A. McPherson, A.M. Galloway, and W. McGhie. Thin plate buckling mitigation and reduction challenges for naval ships. *Journal of Marine Engineering & Technology*, 12(2):3–10, 2013.
7. J.R. Barckhoff. *Total Welding Management American Welding Society with a Product Code of B-AWS-008, USA*, American Welding Society, Miami, Florida, 2005.
8. H. Hemmer, and Ø. Grong. A process model for the heat-affected zone microstructure evolution in duplex stainless-steel weldments: part I. The model. *Metallurgical and Materials Transactions A*, 30(11):2915–2929, 1999.
9. P.L. Jain. *Principles of Foundry Technology.* Tata McGraw-Hill Education, New Delhi, India, 2003.
10. www.foundryinfo-india.org, 2021.
11. Flinn A. Richard. *Fundamentals of Metal Casting.* Addison-Wesley Publishing Company Inc., 1963.
12. C. Gonzalez-Rivera, C. Atlatenco, A. Garcia, M. Ramirez, and D. Universitaria. On the testing of shrinkage tendency of ductile iron prior

to pouring. In *From Conference Proceedings METAL2007 Hradec Nad Moravici TANGER*, 2007.
13. www.askchemicals.com, 2021.
14. www.iitg.ac.in/engfac/ganu/public_html/Metal%20casting%20processes_1.pdf, 2021.
15. F.J. Bradley, S. Heinemann, and J.A. Hoopes. A hydraulics-based/optimization methodology for gating design. *Applied Mathematical Modelling*, 17(8):406–414, 1993.
16. J.P.G. Trancoso, V. Piazza, and E. Frazzon. Simulation-based analysis of additive manufacturing systems for fuel nozzles. *Journal of Aerospace Technology and Management*, 10:4118–4125, 2018.
17. Matthew S. Hoehler, and Rolf Eligehausen. Behavior and testing of anchors in simulated seismic cracks. *ACI Structural Journal*, 105(3):348–357, 2008.
18. W. Mark McGinley. Design of anchor bolts in masonry. *Progress in Structural Engineering and Materials*, 8:155–164, 2006.
19. N. Subramanian. Recent developments in the design of anchor bolts. *The Indian Concrete Journal*, 74: 407–414, 2000.
20. www.i-micronews.com, 2020.
21. A.R. Razali and Y. Qin. *A Review on Micro-Manufacturing, Micro-Forming and Their Key Issues*, Procedia Engineering, Elsevier, Vol. 53, 665–672, 2013.
22. www.marketsandmarkets.com, 2020.
23. S.P. Leo Kumar, J. Jerald, and S. Kumanan. Manufacturing application of micromachining for automobile components. In *Twenty Eighth National Convention of Mechanical Engineers and National Seminar on Emerging Technologies in Product Development for Safe and Sustainable Mobility*, September 3–5, 2012.
24. www.synova.ch, 2020.
25. X. Peng, L. Kong, J.Y.H. Fuh, and H. Wang. A review of post-processing technologies in additive manufacturing. *Journal of Manufacturing and Materials Processing*, 5(2):38, 2021.
26. I. Gibson, D. Rosen, and B.Stucker. Business opportunities and future directions. In *Additive Manufacturing Technologies*, Springer, New York, 2015.
27. N.E. Vaskenly and M. Dhanya. Smart factories: An Indian scenario. *International Journal of Pure and Applied Mathematics*, 118(9):505–509, 2018.
28. J. Ramesh, M. MohanRam, and Y.S. Varadarajan. Sustainable value addition to Micro, Small, and Medium Enterprises (MSMEs) in India: A review of Industry 4.0. *International Journal of Advanced Research in Basic Engineering Sciences and Technology (IJARBEST)*, 5(7):343–350, 2019.
29. P.P. Khargonekar. Future of smart manufacturing in a global economy, 2018, http://faculty.sites.uci.edu/khargonekar/files/2018/05/S.
30. P. Zheng, H. Wang, Z. Sang, R.Y. Zhong, Y. Liu, et al. Smart manufacturing systems for Industry 4.0: conceptual framework, scenarios, and future perspectives. *Front. Mech. Eng.*, Vol. 13, No. 2:137–150, 2018, https://doi.org/10.1007/s11465-018-0499-5.
31. P. Zawadzki, and K. Żywicki. Smart product design and production control for effective mass customization in the Industry 4.0 concept. *Management and Production Engineering Review*, 7(3):105–112, 2016.

32. MTConnect Institute. *MTConnect Standard. Part 1—Overview and Protocol.* Version 1.0.1. 2009. https://static1.squarespace.com/static/54011775e4b0bc1fe0fb8494/t/55800405e4b057 e97372fe59/1434452997276/MTC_Part_1_Overview_v1.0.1R10_02_09.pdf
33. H. Kagermann, J. Helbig, A. Hellinger, et al. Recommendations for implementing the strategic initiative INDUSTRIE 4.0: Securing the future of German manufacturing industry. Final report of the Industrie 4.0 Working Group, Forschungsunion, Germany, 2013.
34. S. Mittal, M.A. Khan, D. Romero and T. Wuest. Building blocks for adopting smart manufacturing. *Procedia Manufacturing*, 34:978–985, 2019, DOI: 10.1016/j.promfg.2019.06.098.
35. M.N.O.Sadiku, O.D. Olaleye, and S.M. Musa. Smart manufacturing: A primer. *International Journal of Trend in Research and Development*, 6(6):9–12, 2019.
36. J.M. Dagadu, and S. Gaikwad. Small scale industry and its present senario in Indian industrilization. *Excel Journal of Engineering Technology and Management Science (An International Multidisciplinary Journal)*, I(5):1–4, 2013.
37. K. Pundir. The role of Industry 4.0 of small and medium enterprises in Uttar Pradesh. *ABS International Journal of Management*, 6(2):68–73, 2018.
38. blog.safetyculture.com, 2020.
39. www.cdc.gov, 2020.
40. www.osha.europa.eu, 2020.
41. www.emilms.fema.gov, 2020.

Chapter 6

Conclusions

The COVID-19 pandemic forced a "change in perspective" for all. It brought in a behavioral change, i.e., concentrating upon a coherent vision, vigor toward cleaning/decontaminating common public places and a renewed emphasis in local manufacturing. This has brought in a golden opportunity for the society to nurture a "collective spirit" against thorough "individualism". Consolidated approaches toward coordination, cooperation and accountability adapted during the recent global pandemic have helped in fortification of sustainable development, accelerating inclusive economic growth and facilitating national integration at unforeseen levels. There is a substantial emphasis upon an economy which in essence has the characteristics of humanism, ecological responsibility, societal upliftment and inclusivity against the sole stress upon pure economics. This has led to entrepreneurship driven by decentralized solutions, manufacturing and creating local level employment. Effort has to be made to support the self-employed and prospective entrepreneurs by providing them with adequate know-how of various technologies so that customized improvements in the technology are encouraged, increasing its operational efficiency, ergonomics, aesthetics and performance. Thus, government organizations might help facilitate accessibility to various resources which include credit, testing facilities, logistics support, new R&D advancements and state-of-the-art infrastructure to prospective entrepreneurs. This approach will consolidate a strong financial stewardship, accountability and transparency in the use of public funds. It will encourage community-based solutions, nourish inclusive economic growth and facilitate the business entities with pilot products, technology and design concepts.

It has been realized that there is a low degree of visibility and awareness of the activities and advancements in R&D laboratories. The solutions, obtained in various public-funded organizations, ought to have an effective impact on the society at large and the investment ought to have the mandated outcomes. Through the years it has been observed that there is a large pool of outstanding students who want to work for the society; however, they lack the requisite technical knowledge in the domain of manufacturing and agriculture, which are the two primary economic drivers for the nation.

DOI: 10.1201/9781003331179-6

It is important that adequate research and investment are directed toward agriculture and manufacturing to aptly tackle a societal crisis such as a pandemic. It is also vital that the youth are engaged in inter-disciplinary domains such as Agrionics, farm mechanization, post-harvest technologies and other agrarian manufacturing domains. Adequate attention through creative modeling and sustainable innovations is required to consolidate the entire value chain. This will also positively boost the agrarian economy and the rural populace. Skill development initiatives for the youth will equip them with adequate skills and prepare them for the impending industrial scenario. It will also plant the seeds of sustainability, innovative temper and analytical bent of mind. Well-knit coordination among the entrepreneurs, universities and R&D institutions will bridge the gap of this skill mismatch, which is one of the root causes of unemployment all over the world. Such a beautiful and balanced academic–entrepreneurial ecosystem will encourage the idea of collaborative thinking.

To increase employment prospects, there is a need to increase decentralization of services through the concept of "eco-civilization system", a valid example of which is decentralized management of wastes. Presently, most of the waste management services are provided by local government institutions. There are existent operational problems such as unskilled sanitation workers, periodic skill upgradation, which consequently reduces sanitation service quality and causes service disruption. A framework of circular economy consisting of biological and technical disposal processes will support this model. Methods to provide innovative waste management services in a safe, efficient and courteous manner, creating environmental sustainability, promoting waste diversion and maintaining a clean city are required. *Sustainable design* can bring to market new products and services with long term social and environmental benefits. Therefore, involving private waste management operating agencies, to whom local governments allocate waste management fees collected from taxpayers, will provide better results. The change toward sustainable and circular business model innovation should integrate elements from macro (global trends and drivers), meso (ecosystem and value cocreation) and micro (company, customers and consumers) levels.

Thus, in a nutshell, it is important to target the root causes of existent socio-ecological problems rather than targeting the effects. It is very important that the micro, small and medium enterprises (MSMEs) are brought into the fold as partners for dissolution of the problems. A robust business opportunity for the entrepreneurial entities will make scaling of production possible in a time-bound manner. This will be the actual realization of the "concept to field" ideology and will be the primary metric of success for the public-funded R&D institutions at large.

Annexure I

Facemask: One of the most important features in facemasks is the hydrophobicity (water repelling nature of mask materials). In order to test the water repelling ability, the wettability test can be performed by measuring the contact angle that the liquid creates at the solid surface of the non-woven polypropylene layer with a specific pore size of the exposed layer of the facemask. The easiest way to measure the contact angle of the mask is to find out the tangent profile at the liquid–solid interface with a 6 μL distilled water droplet on a 0.3 mm thick polypropylene fabric sample surface (Figure AI.1).

The hydrophobicity of any surface is determined by the contact angle >90°. The measured contact angle on most of the polypropylene (PP) mask surfaces is found to be ~125°, which means PP masks can be utilized to avoid the spread of virus. It is important to note that household makeshift masks are often manufactured using cotton cloth/fabric, but the cotton materials have been found to be hydrophilic and may not be suitable for making facemasks under prevalent conditions of the pandemic as the virus may travel through water droplets.

Apart from wettability, the effective pore size of the facemask's surfaces determines the penetration of droplets released during coughing and sneezing. In order to study the pore size and get the information about the distribution of fibers, field-emission scanning electron microscopy (FESEM) of samples can be analyzed (Figure AI.2). FESEM images of PP layers of different pore size ranges of (a) >100 μm, (b) 55 ± 5 μm and (c) 35 ± 5 μm are given in Figure AI.2.

Reusability of mask PP materials can be compared with the cotton facemasks. It has been found that after first wash, the polypropylene cloth gets stretched, marginally increasing the pore size from 35 ± 5 μm to 40 ± 5 μm, and thereafter, it remains constant even after three washes. Microstructures of PP fabric after (a) 1st wash and (b) 3rd wash and cotton fabric after (c) 1st wash and (d) 3rd wash are given in Figure AI.3. Tearing of fibers could

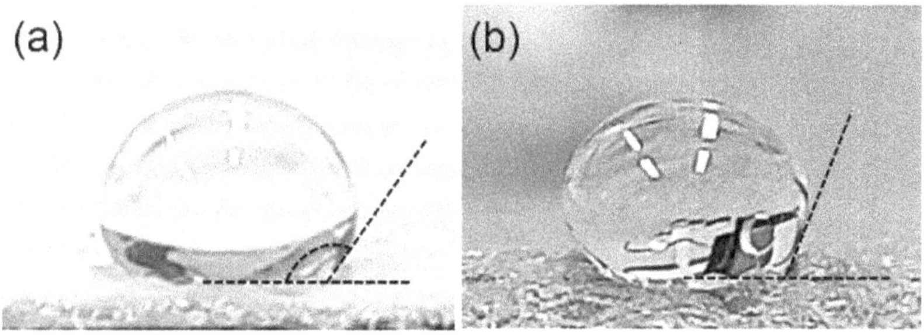

Figure AI.1 Contact angle measurement on the surface of (a) non-woven polypropylene and (b) commercially available N95 facemasks.

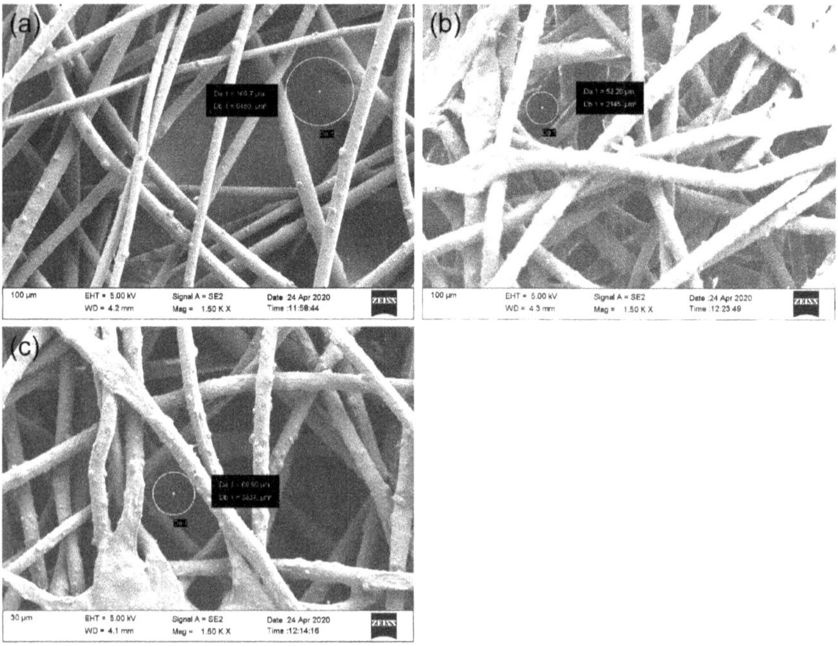

Figure AI.2 FESEM images of PP layers of different pore size ranges of (a) >100 µm, (b) 55 ± 5 µm and (c) 35 ± 5 µm.

be observed after the third wash (Figure AI.3d). This reveals the fact that PP fabric can be reused for a longer duration compared to cotton masks.

The anticipation of enhancement of pore size due to the insertion of needles and cotton threads can be analyzed by examination of the FESEM image, as shown in Figure AI.4. This image clearly indicates that there is no evidence of pore size enhancement in the stitched region.

To ensure the fact that the developed mask is capable enough to prevent bioaerosols, i.e., aerosols containing bacteria and viruses, bacterial

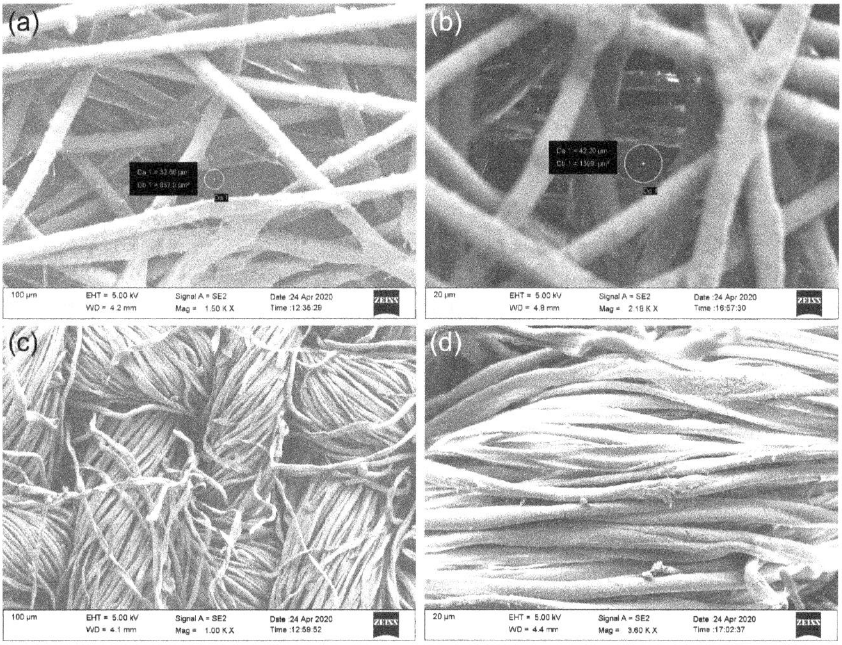

Figure AI.3 PP vs. cotton fabric: microstructure of PP fabric after (a) 1st wash and (b) 3rd wash and cotton fabric after (c) 1st wash and (d) 3rd wash.

filtration efficiency (BFE) as per the *ASTM standard F2101* should be studied. Furthermore, the particulate filter efficiency (PFE) tests as per standard ASTM F2299 must be carried out as a quality indicator for the manufactured facemasks. The performance of the developed mask based on the report received from the South India Textile Research Association (SITRA) is tabulated in **Table AI.1**. The test reports clearly illustrate high efficiency of the facemasks, with the bacterial filtration efficiency as high as 99.9% and particulate filtration efficiency as high as 95.46% along with good breathability (measured as pressure loss using the MS 36954C standard) and splash resistance (as per ASTM 1862) against synthetic blood.

Hydraulic variant disinfection walkway: The "hydraulic variant disinfection walkway" is a spraying system designed for sanitizing every individual before entering into main entrance gates of offices, hospitals, market premises [see ref. 14 of Chapter 2], shopping complexes, housing societies, apartments, railway stations, etc., where movement of a large number of people occurs and there is more chance of spreading infections. The front and side views of the disinfectant mist sprayer pathway are provided in Figure AI.5. The main elements of the disinfectant walkway are: fans, sensors, spraying nozzles along with the chemical storage tank and a centrifugal pump. The pathway has a width of 1.50 m and a length of 2.40 m. Two

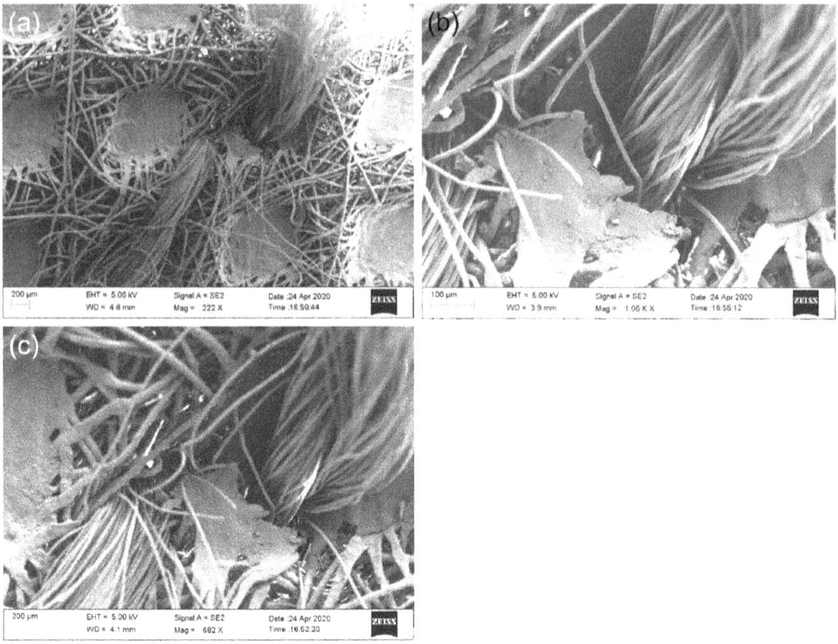

Figure AI.4 Microstructures of the stitched region showing no apparent increase in pore size.

Table AI.1 Performance of the developed facemasks based on the test reports from SITRA

Sl.	*Tests/Standards*	*Results*
1.	**Bacterial filtration efficiency (ASTM F 2101)** Test organisms used: Staphylococcus aureus ATCC 6538 mean particle size of challenging aerosol: 3.0 ± 0.3 μm Flow rate of aerosol: 28.5 L/min	99.9%
2.	**Particulate filtration efficiency at 0.3 microns (ASTM F2299/F2299M-03 (2010))**	95.46%
3.	**Differential pressure (IS 16289:2014 Annexure C)**	43.0 Pa/cm^2
4.	**Splash resistance (ASTM F1862/F1862M-13)** at 160 mmHg	Pass
5.	**Flammability (16 CFR Part-1610)**	Class 1

nozzles are used from opposite sides with 2.5 bar of pressure to ensure effective delivery of the disinfecting mist. To ensure optimum coverage of sanitizer over every person, four wall-mounted fans of 9-inch diameter and 250 rpm capacity are used from corners of the pathway for spreading of mists. The system comes with two numbers of embedded non-contact type

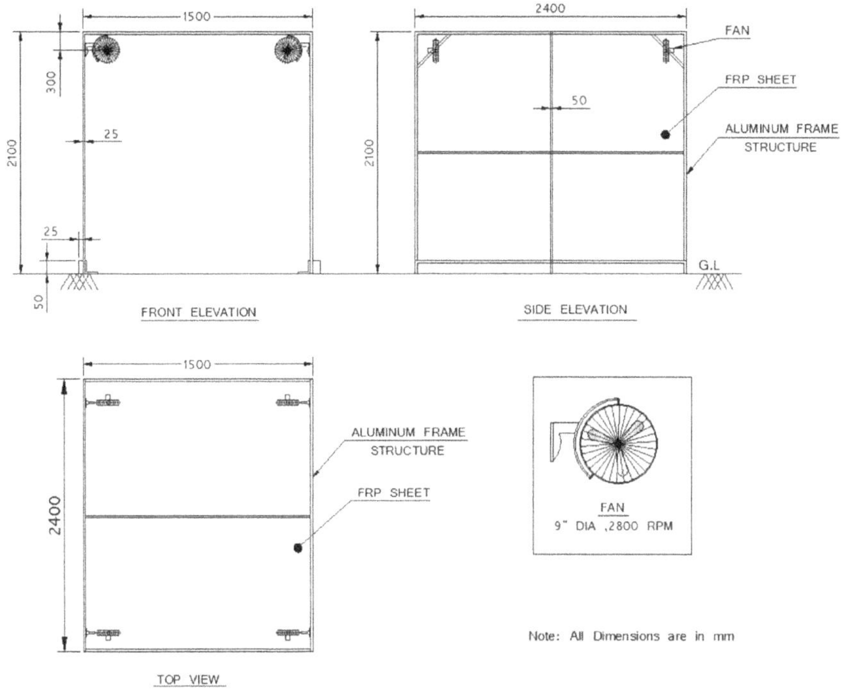

Figure AI.5 Front, side and top views of the disinfectant mist sprayer pathway.

sensors with one controller unit and a timer for switching on and off the system. The system can also run non-stop bypassing the sensor system during entry of more persons at the start of shift duty.

The disinfectant mist sprayer pipeline diagram is represented in Figure AI.6. The technical configuration of the unit is given in **Table AI.2**, and the technical details of the system are represented in **Table AI.3**.

Pneumatic variant disinfection walkway: The disinfectant walkway is made of acrylic transparent sheets fixed with aluminum frames. The approximate overall dimension of the system is 1.2–1.5 m (L) × 2.2–2.5 m (H) × 1.0 m (W). The roof is made of non-metallic corrugated sheets. Figure AI.7 shows the developed pneumatic variant disinfection walkway. The developed sensor-based disinfection walkway has the feature of contactless operation which is very important in pandemic situations. Any object entering into the walkway will be detected by an infrared (IR)-based proximity sensor placed in the entry side of the chamber and enables the non-contact type switch to start and stop the spray automatically. Two double-phase internal mixing nozzles are used for spraying the air-water mist. Entry and exit sides of the chamber are open. There are two double-phase internal mixing nozzles placed in the exit side of the chamber focusing toward the center of the chamber. The nozzles are fixed in such a way

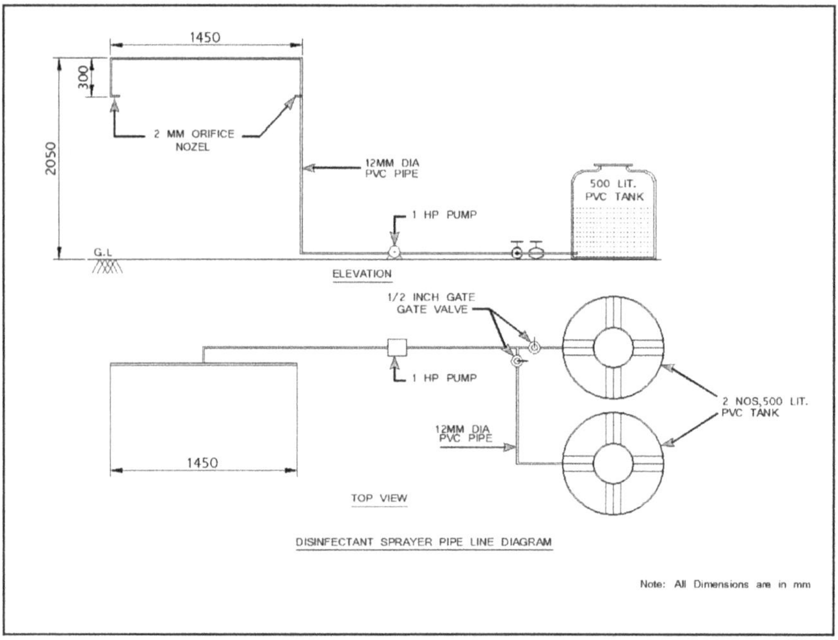

Figure AI.6 Disinfectant mist sprayer pipeline diagram.

Table AI.2 Technical configuration of the hydraulic variant disinfection walkway

Hydraulic pump capacity:	I hp
Line pressure:	5 bar
Tank capacity:	500 L
No. of nozzles:	2 Nos.
Fans:	4 Nos., 9-inch dia., 250 rpm
Spray mixture:	As per guidelines issued by the "Health and Family Welfare Department", Government of W.B. or any other appropriate authority

that one is oriented toward the upper side and other is oriented toward the lower side. Presently, the spraying time is fixed at 20 sec. However, the spraying time can be adjusted as per requirement. The schematic diagram of pneumatic variant disinfection is given in Figure AI.8.

Pneumatically operated mobile indoor disinfection (POMID) unit: The POMID unit [see ref. 19 of Chapter 2] may be used for removal, deactivation or killing of pathogenic microorganisms present inside a closed chamber like rooms, halls, building corridors using water/other liquids mixed with chemical disinfectants. The compressed air is used to form mist/jet spray of liquid disinfectants to sanitize the indoor area. This unit

Table AI.3 Technical details of the hydraulic variant disinfection system development

Design of the disinfectant pathway:	The dimension of the glass fixed-aluminum framed disinfectant pathway is about 2.4 m long and 1.5 m wide with height of 2.1 m. The disinfectant pathway is covered with glass reinforced polyester translucent fiber glass sheets fixed in aluminum frames from both sides. The roof is covered with fibre reinforced plastic (FRP) sheets.
Pumping and spraying unit:	A 1 hp centrifugal pump with a PVC pipe network is used for spraying the disinfectant connected through the 300 L capacity PVC tank at the ground level. Two numbers of vortex type small orifice misting nozzles are used from both the sides at a height of 1.6 m from the ground level as shown in the 2-D drawing. Fluid flows through the small orifice of the nozzles at a pressure of 2.5 bar, which creates sufficient turbulence to atomize the water into a fine fog. Four numbers of 9-inch diameter fans with a rotational speed of 2800 rpm are mounted at the four corners of the disinfectant chamber directed toward the nozzles. Disinfectant ejected from the orifice in a full cone pattern rapidly breaks down into a homogeneous fog due to the turbulence of air created by the fans.
Sensors and controller:	At the point of the pathway, two numbers of non-contact type sensors are fixed at a height of 1.2 m with one controller and timer to detect the movement of any person through the disinfectant chamber.
Disinfection process:	The disinfectant chamber is fully controlled by an electrically operated pump, non-contact type sensors, a controller and a timer. When a person enters into the chamber, the electrically operated pump starts and disinfectant fluid is sprayed through the orifice of the nozzles followed by the mist formation due to the turbulence generated by the fans positioned at the four corners of the pathway. The mist spray is calibrated for 10 sec to 40 sec of spraying and then stops automatically until the next person enters into the chamber.

is mounted on a four-wheel trolley to make it movable. The system comprises a pneumatic compressor system, two storage tanks for two different disinfectants and spray systems with mopping facility (Figures AI.9). The pneumatic compressor, maintained at 6–8 bar pressure, ensures optimum mist formation from two different disinfectant liquids during the indoor sanitization process. The spray system has nozzles, located in two tiers, in addition to a hand-held flexible nozzle. This system is designed to sanitize the floor by the spray nozzles located in the lower tier, the upper tier nozzles are meant for the purpose of disinfecting the beds, tables, etc. The spray angle of lower tier nozzles is adjustable along the horizontal plane and the top tier nozzles are adjustable both in horizontal and vertical directions. The hand-held flexible spray arm can be used for disinfecting in any other places as per requirement. The system is also equipped with mopping facility to mop the floor in order to soak the liquid disinfectants, if any, from the floor. The advantage of the system is that the particle size could be as small as 100 micron and the operating cost is much less, owing to less usage of disinfectant liquids. Figure AI.10 shows the flow diagram of the POMID

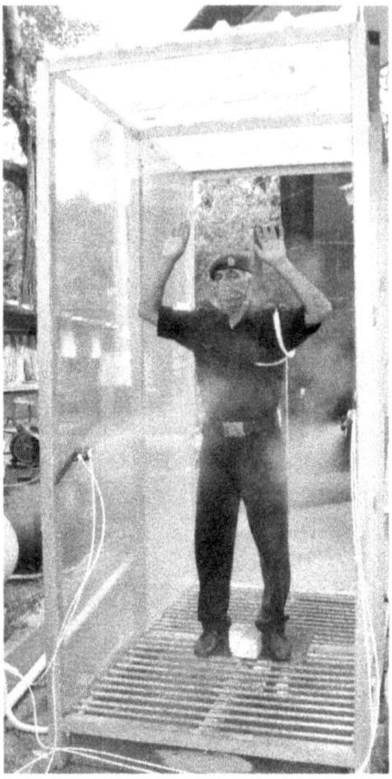

Figure AI.7 Developed pneumatic variant disinfection walkway.

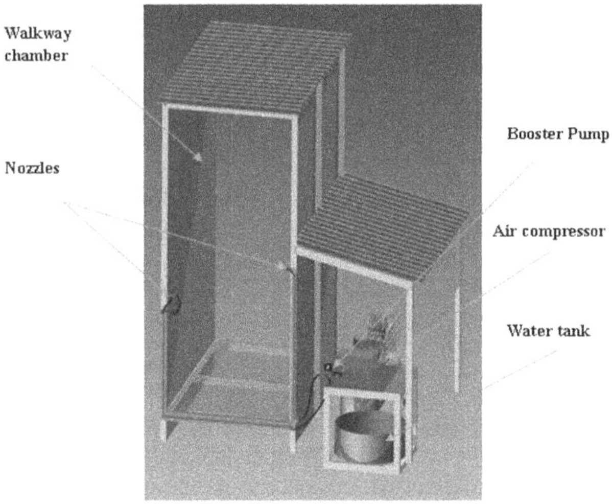

Figure AI.8 Schematic diagram of the pneumatic variant disinfection walkway.

unit. Figure AI.11 displays the prototype and demonstration of the POMID unit.

Solar-based intelligent mask ATM-cum-thermal scanner (IntelliMAST): Intelligent mask ATM-cum-thermal scanner (IntelliMAST), an AI-based intelligent machine identifies the person with or without facemask. An

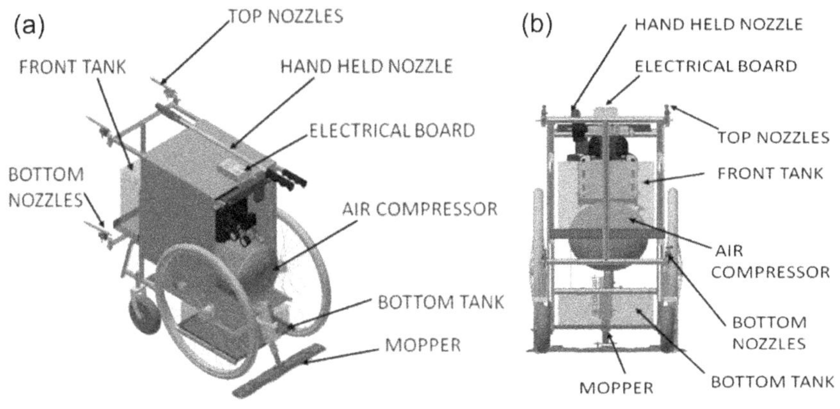

Figure AI.9 Isometric and rear views of the POMID unit.

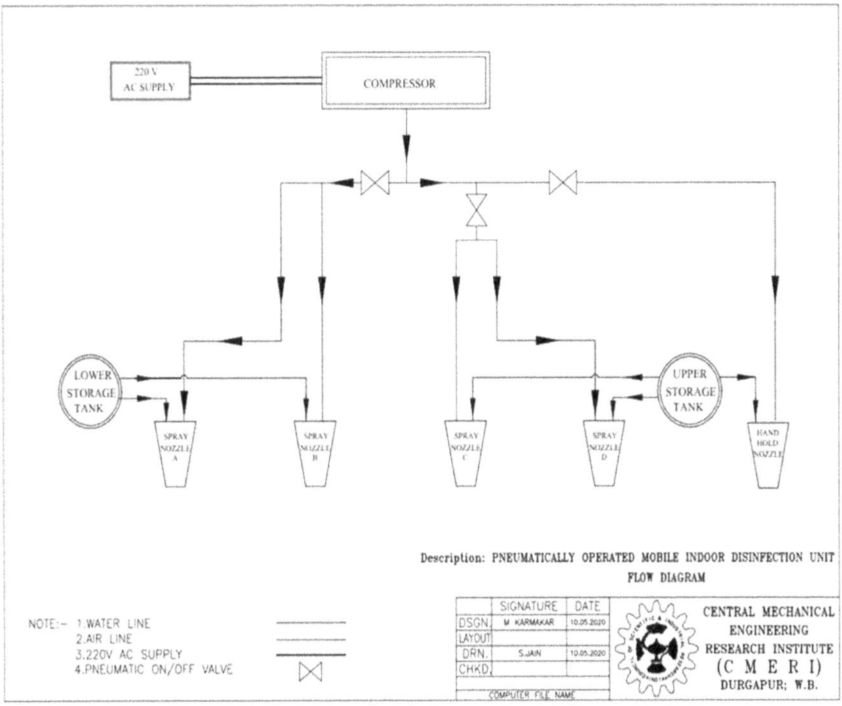

Figure AI.10 Flow diagram of POMID.

automatic IR-based thermal scanning mechanism of IntelliMAST takes person's body temperature for deciding whether he/she should get entry in the institution or not. The machine, in the first phase, detects the person coming in its proximity and checks forehead temperature using an IR-based thermal sensor. If the system finds the body temperature of the person

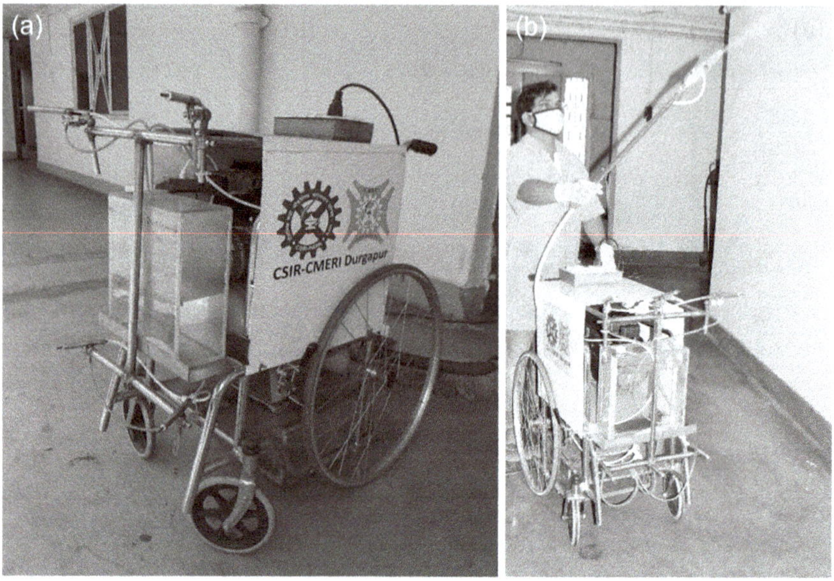

Figure AI.11 The POMID unit.

higher than the permissible limit, it raises an audio-visual alarm otherwise it enters into the second phase of the scanning process and the system takes a photograph of the person using a built-in camera. The computer vision is used to identify the facial feature of the person. The detected facial feature is then fed to an AI engine equipped with the pretrained deep learning model (trained for classifying masked and non-masked face with higher than 98% precision). If the system detects that the person's face is classified (with a confidence higher than the predefined threshold) as a masked face, it prompts the person as "Admitted" with lighting up a green light signal mounted on the system. However, if the system classifies the person's face as a non-masked face, it triggers an audio-visual alarm and enters into the third phase. In the third phase, the system prompts for I-Card of the person and if machine detects a valid I-Card, it activates the facemask ATM mechanism of the IntelliMAST. The facemask ATM mechanism then starts operating and dispenses one set of facemask to the person, records his photograph and sends the person's information in the form an e-mail to the predefined authority(ies) of the institution for payment settlement. The IntelliMAST is designed to be deployed in the outdoor environment and powered with an integrated solar setup and electrical grid for 24×7 operations.

The system also comprises open-source graphical user interface (GUI) software for controlling all the above three phases of the system, raising an audio-visual alarm and a user interface for live feedback through

"Admitted" or "Not Admitted" on-screen message display. The system can be integrated with any access control system for operating turnstile, barrier gate or can be customized to act as touchless attendance system. The image of the IntelliMAST is shown at Figure AI.12 and the labeled sketch of the solar-powered unit is given in Figure AI.13. The specification of the system is given in Table AI.4. The process flow chart indicating working of IntelliMAST is represented in Figure AI.14.

Touchless faucet (TouF): washbasin-mounted contactless soap-cum-water dispensing unit: The touchless faucet can be developed to cater the frequent need of washing hands with soap and water. The faucet can be very easily mounted by replacing the existing tap of any washbasin. This system dispenses water 30 seconds after dispensing soap in a touch free mechanism. When a person approaches the sensor on the basin-mounted touchless faucet, a predefined amount of soap (few milliliters) will be dispensed from the tap, momentarily. After rubbing hand for 30 seconds, clean water is dispensed from the same tap. The arrangement aims to reduce wastage of water and is suited for homes and offices. The system also works manually in case of power failure. That is, the faucet may be used manually by operating the knob provided on the left side wall of the faucet. Figure AI.15 shows the developed touchless faucet (TouF): washbasin-mounted contactless soap-cum-water dispensing unit. The specifications of the system are given in **Table AI.5**. Block schematic of operation of the touchless faucet is represented in Figure AI.16.

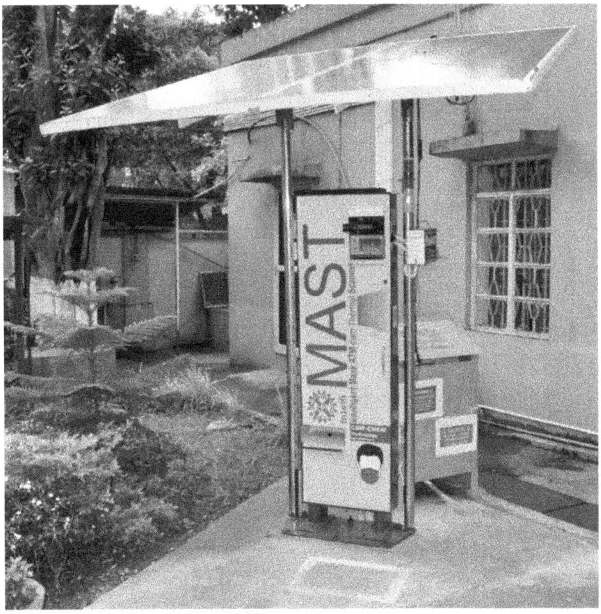

Figure AI.12 Developed solar-based intelligent mask ATM-cum-thermal scanner.

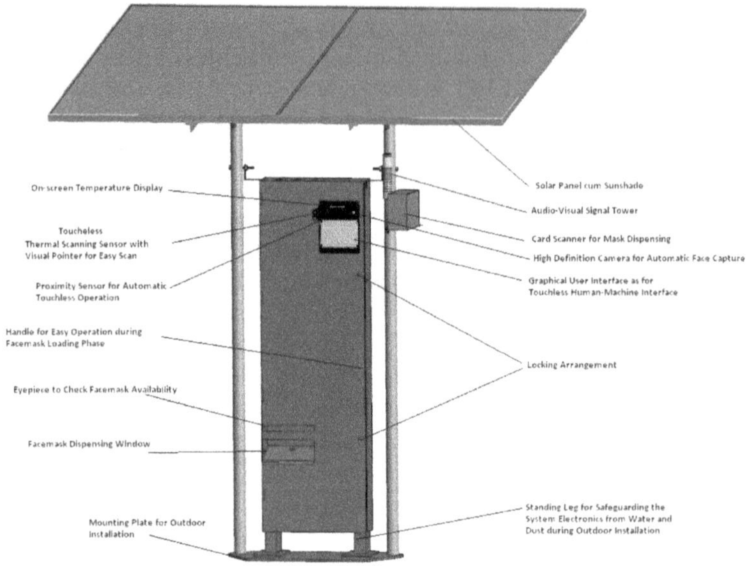

Figure AI.13 Labeled sketch of solar-powered IntelliMAST.

Dry fogging shoe disinfector (DFSD): Various studies suggest that virus spread occurs from the soles of shoes [see ref. 13 of Chapter 2]. The shoe soles of medical staff act as virus carriers; therefore, disinfection of shoe soles before walking out of hospital wards is recommended. The dry fogging shoe disinfector (DFSD) atomizes water-based disinfectants into very fine size (<10 micron) particles to ensure that the number of particles cluster around the pathogens stuck on the shoe sole and enables higher contact time of the disinfectant with the microorganisms present. The smaller size of the particles also guarantees minimum wetting of the surfaces and no damage of shoe leather/Rexine material. Technical specifications of the DFSD are provided in **Table AI.6.**

Figure AI.17 shows the developed DFSD and schematic diagram of the system is given in Figure AI.18.

360° car flusher: The 360° car flusher [see ref. 23 of Chapter 2] is developed for sanitization of cars, trucks, buses, etc. The sanitizing system can be used in long stretches of highways, vicinity of markets, shopping malls, office campuses as well as residential complexes, etc. The active sensor-based automatic power supply to pump is used in this technology. Hence, no manual intervention is required to operate the pump.

A piping network with distributed spraying nozzles mounted around the pipe network can be designed. The active sensors are placed before the sanitizing unit to detect the vehicle and subsequently supply of power to the

Table AI.4 Specifications of the IntelliMAST

Specification:	**AI-based facemask scanning system:**	• Precision in detection of mask on the human face: >98%. • The deep learning (DL) model improves continuously based on the collected data. • Equipped with over-the-air (OTA) programming and update feature. • IoT-based design for intimation of non-masked person through the Internet. • An open-source machine learning platform used for model training. • Human–computer interaction: graphical user interface (GUI).
	Facemask ATM:	• Mask carrying capacity: 25 slots for loading 25 packets (each can contain four facemasks). • I-Card-based mask dispensing: any barcode based I-Card shall work (registration needed). • Closed-loop hardware-based controller for precise quantity control. • Maintenance-free dispensing coil mechanism.
	Contactless thermal scanning:	• Technology: IR-based thermal sensor. • Operation: automatic • Accuracy: $\pm 1^\circ$C. • Measurement resolution: 0.02°C.
	Power system:	• Type: hybrid power (solar + grid). • Total system load = ~50 W. • Continuous operation = 10 hours (only on solar), 24 hours (on hybrid power).
	In-built disinfection:	• Built-in UV-C light for auto-disinfection of mask packets and other inanimate surfaces. • 10-minute auto-cut operation.
	Modular design:	• Can be integrated with any access control system like fully automatic vertical tripod turnstile, flap turnstile or barrier gate. • Can be customized as touchless I-Card-based attendance system.
Usage:	It is essential to wear the facemask whenever visiting public places. Sometimes, due to personal mistake an employee may forget to come up with the facemask and requires a mask, in that situation this system provides all help. The system can be integrated with a touchless entry system for the offices, residential complexes, shopping malls, etc.	
Key features:	• Intelligent detection of persons with facemask or without facemask. • I-Card-based facemask dispensing mechanism along with close-loop electronic controller circuitry. • Automatic thermal scanner for taking body temperature. • High intensity audio-visual alarm for public awareness. • Integrated solar power set up for standalone operation. • Auto-controlled built-in UV-C light for auto-disinfection of mask packets and other inanimate surfaces and 10-minute auto-cut operation. • Can be customized as a touchless access control mechanism with flap gates/turnstiles/barrier gates. • Audio-visual tower type (LED) alarm system.	

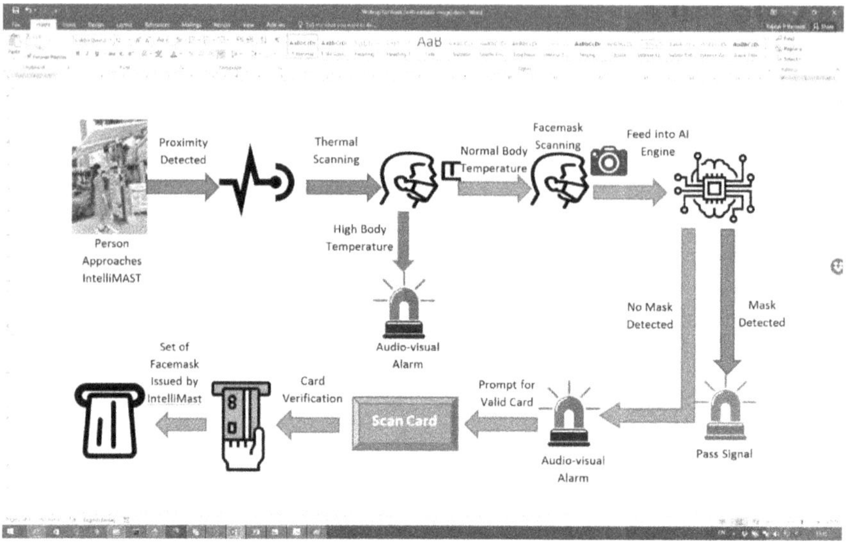

Figure AI.14 Process flow chart indicating working of IntelliMAST.

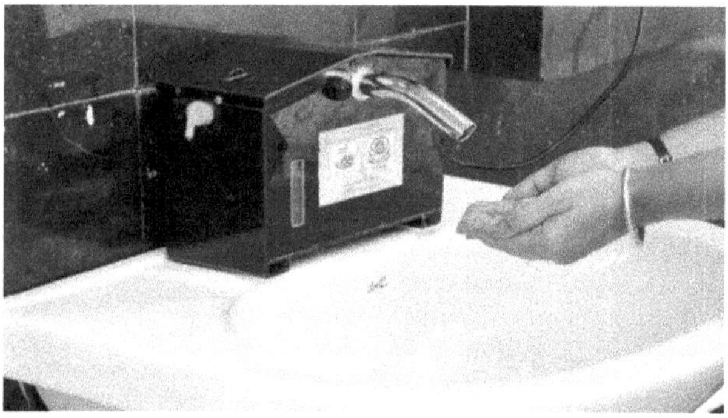

Figure AI.15 Developed touchless faucet (TouF): washbasin-mounted contactless soap-cum-water dispensing unit.

pump is switched on and the spray system starts immediately. The vehicle passes through the sanitizing unit and gets sanitized immediately and after crossing the vehicle, the pumps are switched off immediately. This system needs mainly a normal water tank and a high-pressure pump to spray disinfectant mixed with water all around the running vehicles for vehicle sanitization. The automatic spraying on the vehicle is done by the use of a through beam sensor unit. The sensor unit consists of a set of an infrared (IR) transmitter and IR receiver module. The IR transmitter module generates a continuous stream of IR signal at 38 KHz, radiated from a low beam

Table AI.5 Novelty of the touchless faucet (TouF): washbasin-mounted contactless soap-cum-water dispensing unit

Novelty of the system:	Dual mode operation (automatic and manual-in-of-power failure)	
	Basin mounted	
	Single tap dispenser for soap as well as water	
	Single IR sensor for both soap and water	
	Minimal water usage	
	Plug and use	
	Material used:	1. 1.Acrylic (more attractive)
		Powder-coated steel (more durable)
	Dimensions:	250 × 115 × 215 mm

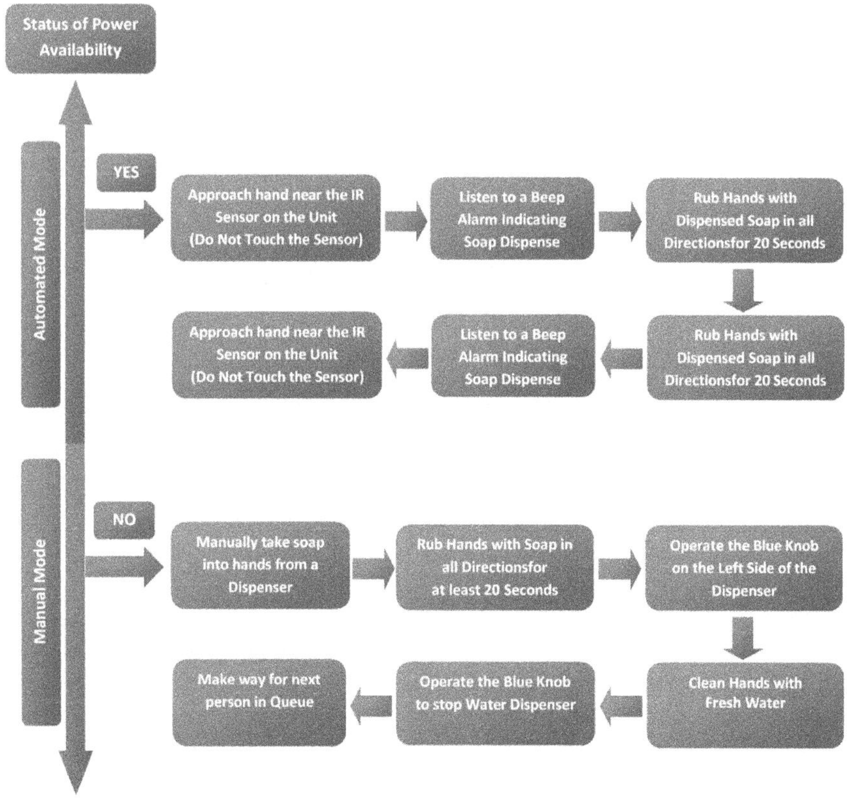
Status of Power Availability
Automated Mode
YES
Approach hand near the IR Sensor on the Unit (Do Not Touch the Sensor)
Listen to a Beep Alarm Indicating Soap Dispense
Rub Hands with Dispensed Soap in all Directionsfor 20 Seconds
Approach hand near the IR Sensor on the Unit (Do Not Touch the Sensor)
Listen to a Beep Alarm Indicating Soap Dispense
Rub Hands with Dispensed Soap in all Directionsfor 20 Seconds
Manual Mode
NO
Manually take soap into hands from a Dispenser
Rub Hands with Soap in all Directionsfor at least 20 Seconds
Operate the Blue Knob on the Left Side of the Dispenser
Make way for next person in Queue
Operate the Blue Knob to stop Water Dispenser
Clean Hands with Fresh Water

Figure AI.16 Block Schematic of operation of the touchless faucet.

angle IR light-emitting diode (LED), controlled by a pulse width modulator (PWM) generator. The IR receiver module has an IR receiver integrated circuit (IC), which receives the IR signal sent from the IR transmitted module. A controller IC of the receiver module captures the signal from the

Table AI.6 Technical specifications and usage of the developed dry fogging shoe disinfector

Technical specifications:	Material	Stainless steel
	Diameter of piezoceramics	20 mm
	Atomizing quantity	~5000 mL/h
	Water level	40–80 mm
	Working voltage	48 V DC
	Current	4.6–5 A
	Power:	350 W
	Battery (for DC operated)	12 V 32 AH
	SMPS (for AC operated)	230 V 10 A
	Back-up time (battery operated)	3–4 hours for single charging
Usage:	Shoe sole, electronic equipment, cabin of vehicles, clean rooms, hospitals	
Competing features:	• The dry fogging system generates microdroplets with particle size in the range of 0.1 to 10 microns. The particles smaller size of remain suspended in air for significant periods of time. This results in increased penetration and diffusion of the disinfectant in the air, and as a result, the contact time with microorganisms increases. The surfaces also do not get wet. • System can be operated both with grid supply (AC mode) and battery bank power supply (DC mode). • Size and number density of microdroplets can be controlled through adjustment of the depth of the water level in the disinfector tank resulting in a greater area of coverage of the droplets. • Reservoir filter to prevent the entry of any foreign solid particles in the disinfector tank thereby enhancing the life of the atomizing plate. • Unique on–off feature to protect the atomizing plate from dry run, in case the level of disinfection fluid in the reservoir falls below a preset value.	

IR receiver IC and determines the presence or absence of any vehicle. The controller turns on a Normally Open (NO) contact type relay once the presence of a vehicle is detected and switches on the pump immediately, thereby starting the spray of sanitizer liquid. Once the vehicle leaves the sanitizer unit, the IR receiver module gets back the IR beam to determine the absence of vehicle and the controller switches off the relay and thereby turning off the pump with a certain delay. This delay time can be adjusted through a potentiometer connected with the controller from 0 to 10 seconds. The sensor unit is powered by 230 V AC.

The electric motor operated high pressure and low flow pump is powered from the electric power supply. The pump and motor are coupled through the belt pulley arrangements. The pump operates at the prescribed rotational speed. The suction side of the pump is connected with a water tank

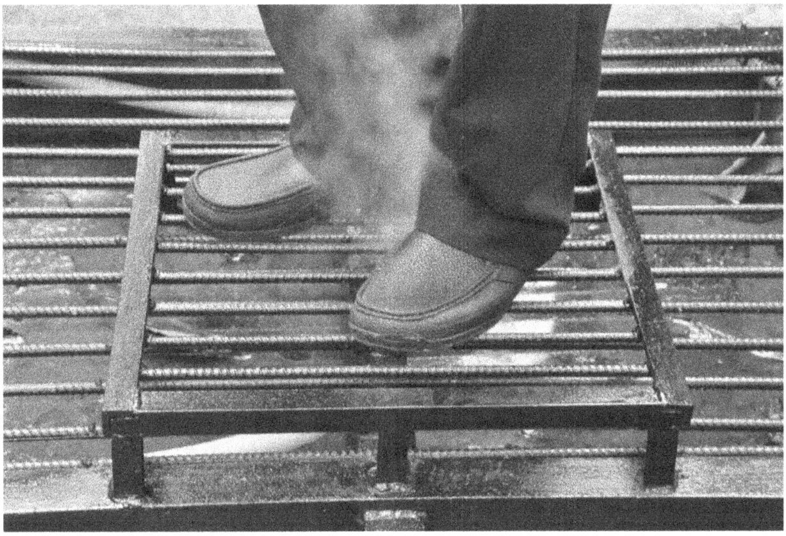

Figure AI.17 Developed dry fogging shoe disinfector.

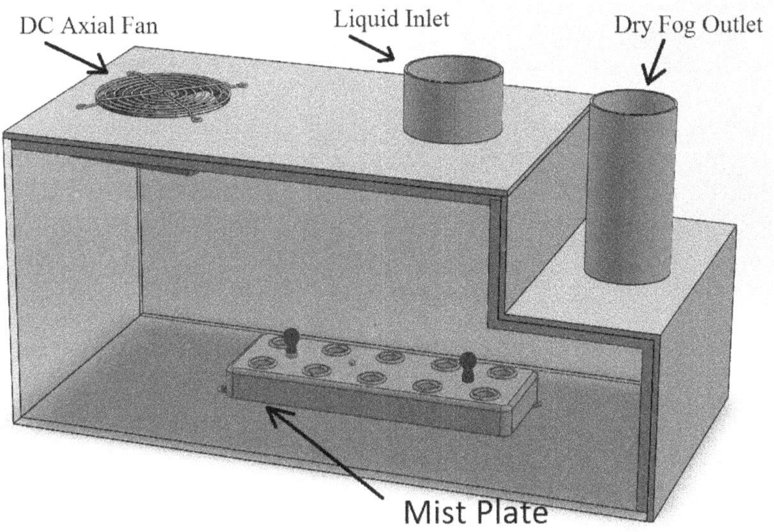

Figure AI.18 Schematic diagram of the dry fogging shoe disinfector.

through the hose pipe. The pump discharge is connected to one side of the pipe network with a flexible hose. The pipe network consists of four 1-inch diameter pipes connected with one by one in a rectangular shape. This rectangular shape pipe network is supported by the Tee type angle arrangements in such a way that the pipe network can be placed properly and there

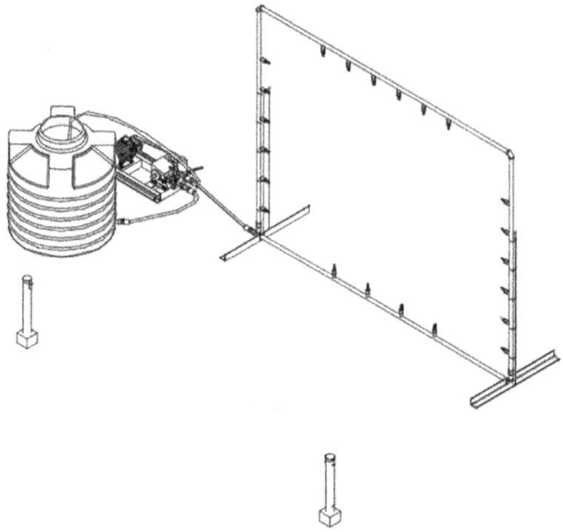

Figure AI.19 Schematic diagram of the 360° car flusher.

are no chances of falling down. There are a total of 20 nozzles attached in the pipe network to spray properly all around the vehicle. The provision is made to sanitize the bottom side of the vehicle by placing four numbers of nozzles in the bottom of the pipe network. These nozzles with pipe are placed in such a way that there is no scope of breaking either the nozzle or the pipe due to vehicle load. Figure AI.19 shows the schematic diagram of the 360° car flusher.

Annexure II

WASTEWATER PURIFICATION TECHNOLOGIES

Various methodologies have been used since the 20th century for municipal wastewater treatment to control water contaminations (e.g., harmful heavy metals, total coliform, fecal coliform) and provide sustainable solutions for the usage in communities for household and agricultural purposes. The reuse of industrial wastewater, in which the effluents are discharged by industry plants, is out of the scope of this book. The present subheading describes use of municipal wastewater, which is a combination of sewer or sanitary sewer generated by domestic uses of water and contains feces or urine from people's toilets, several pathogens, bacteria, metals, etc. In other words, the municipal water consists mostly of gray water (water from sinks, bathtubs, bathrooms, showers, washing machines), black water (water combined with human waste, which is flushed away), soaps and detergents and toilet paper.

Chlorination: Chlorine in its various forms is considered to be a powerful pathogen disinfectant. Sodium hypochlorite (NaOCl which on its reaction with water forms hypochlorous acid and sodium hydroxide) is the most commonly used chlorination bleach in wastewater treatment plants. The hypochlorous acid is a weak acid, while sodium hydroxide is a strong base and thereby upon addition of sodium hypochlorite to water, the pH of water increases. The chemical reaction can be illustrating as follows:

$$2NaOCl + 2H_2O \rightarrow 2NaOH + HOCl + OCl^- + H^+$$

Often ammonia is present in wastewater, which readily reacts with chlorine in the water and gets converted into different chloroamines, like monochloramine, dichloramine and trichloramine. Such chloramines itself act as disinfectants and help to remove many microorganisms. It is believed that the exposure of sunlight degrades NaOCl and liberates free chlorine, which disinfects microorganisms including bacteria and viruses effectively. The chlorination reaction with various organic compounds also leads to the formation of different dissolved organic compounds, which must be filtered off later with an activated carbon filter. Nevertheless, the post treatment after chlorination is highly desirable not only to remove the organic byproduct but also to decrease the concentration of chlorine in water by the dechlorination process. Such dechlorination process involves proper aeration of water and filtration of water through activated carbon filters.

Activated carbon filtration: Activated carbon being highly porous with a high surface area is considered to be one of the most powerful adsorbents to be used for water filtration. The mechanism [1] lies in the physical attractive forces binding solute molecules by van der Waals forces avoiding any chemical interaction. Such binding forces [2] are good enough to trap various organic as well as inorganic compounds effectively. The extent of adsorption depends much on the particle size, pore size and overall surface area. The commercially available activated carbons are categorized in different grades based on their particle size or surface area values mostly in between 500 and 1500 m^2/g. While powdered activated carbon usually contains very fine particles of size range 1–150 μm, granular activated carbon (GAC) has the particle size range of 0.5–4 mm and extruded activated carbon consists of particles of 0.8–4 mm size. It is obvious that smaller the particle size, higher will be the surface area and so the water filtration will be more effective. To achieve high-quality activated carbon, the precursors in the form of coal or biomass must undergo hydrolysis and chemical activation at high temperature. Moreover, contact time is another very important parameter to design the carbon filtration bed. To maintain a particular flow rate the following calculations are useful to design the filtration bed:

$$\text{Linear velocity}\left(m/h\right) = \frac{\text{Flow rate}\left(\frac{m^3}{h}\right)}{\text{Surface area}\left(m^2\right)}$$

$$\text{Contact time}\left(min\right) = \frac{\text{Carbon volume}\left(m^3\right) \times 60\left(\frac{min}{h}\right)}{\text{Flow rate}\left(\frac{m^3}{h}\right)}$$

Based on the abovementioned equation, it is understandable that higher the surface area, lower will be the required carbon volume, thereby shortening the contact time. This indicates that the quality of activated carbon must be very carefully chosen, based on the impurities in the form of suspended solids and colloidal materials present in the water. While for drinking water purification techniques a very high-quality activated carbon is desired, in case of wastewater treatment mostly granular activated carbons (GACs) are utilized to avoid clogging by a wide variety of impurities.

Other than colloidal particles as impurities, activated carbon also removes free chlorine, chloramines and other dissolved organic compounds, present at low concentrations, by effectively adsorbing them from water. The free chlorine, in the form of hypochlorous acid, reacts with activated carbon to form an oxide on the carbon surface [3]. The used activated carbon may further be reactivated by the treatment with high-pressure steam. Such a process includes sterilization through steaming followed by sodium hydroxide to regenerate active sites. Figure AII.1 shows adsorption on activated carbon media. To increase the number of jobs at the local level a cost-effective technique to produce considerably high surface area activated carbon from biomass wastes, like dry leaves, grasses, straw, etc., can be used. Such initiatives will provide a much-needed solution to the agro waste management and generate economic utilization of waste for wastewater treatment.

Floating capsule-based biofilm reactor (FCBBR) methodology: The FCBBR is a hybridized biological treatment technique, adopting the best features of both the activated sludge process along with those of the biofilter process. The aim of installation of the "floating capsule-based biofilm reactor" (FCBBR) is to remove soluble pollutants into harmless metabolites such as carbon dioxide, biomass. This would in turn reduce the BOD/COD level [4]. The FCBBR system retains slow growing microorganisms such as nitrifiers in the form of biofilm. These nitrifiers have the efficiency to reduce the concentration of inorganic nitrogen such as NH_4^+, NO_3^- and

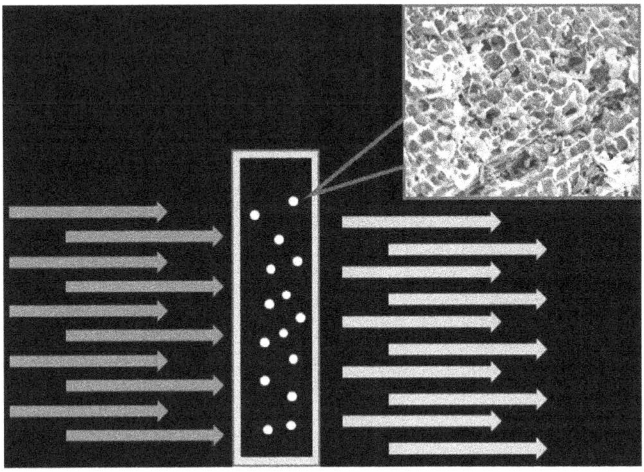

Figure AII.1 Adsorption on activated carbon media.

NO_2^- at a quality rate from the wastewater by nitrification and denitrification processes.

$$\text{Nitrification } NH_{4^+} \xrightarrow{\text{Slow}} NO_{2^-} \xrightarrow{\text{Fast}} NO_{3^-};$$

$$\text{Denitrification Nitrate}(NO_{3^-}) \xrightarrow{\text{Fast}} \text{Nitrite}(NO_{2^-})$$

$$\rightarrow \text{Nitrous oxide } (N_2O) \xrightarrow{\text{Slow}} N_2.$$

Nitrification is a biological oxidation process to oxidize ammonium into nitrite by ammonia-oxidizing bacteria (AOB) then followed by oxidation of nitrite into nitrate by nitrite-oxidizing bacteria (NOB) under aerobic conditions. Denitrification is a biological process that takes place under anaerobic conditions to reduce the oxidized products of nitrogen into their gaseous forms that are released into the air and are mainly nitrous oxide (NO_2) and nitrogen gas (N_2). The advantageous features for the FCBBR process over other biological wastewater treatment systems are given below as:

I. The FCBBR uses biological carriers for biofilm growth as a media so that it can be kept in suspension as shown in Figure AII.2.
II. Continuous flow through process – No need of backwash. Less head loss.
III. Very simple and flexible system of multiple treatments such as BOD, COD removal, nitrification and denitrification.
IV. No need of sludge separation as most of the active biomass is retained along with the biofilm carriers.

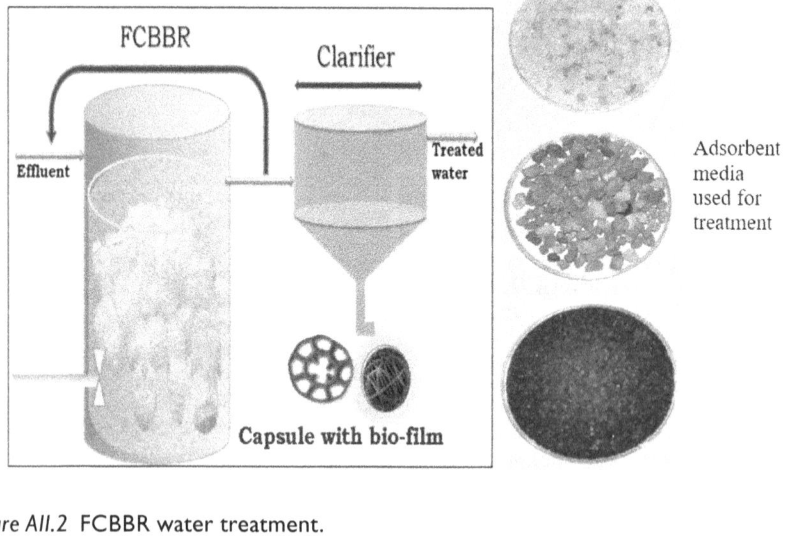

Figure AII.2 FCBBR water treatment.

UV treatment: In the final stage, the treated water is exposed to UV irradiation, especially to deal with any DNA- or RNA-based viruses or bacteria present in the water. The UV-C light with a wavelength of 200–280 nm can effectively damage nucleic acids including DNA and RNA of sporozoites. In the case of bacteria and viruses, UV light inactivates (especially 264 nm) the bacteria from dividing and forming colonies. Different doses are required to inactivate different microorganisms. Although a UV-C dose of 2000–8000 $\mu W.s/cm^2$ is enough to inactivate most of the bacteria and viruses, in some cases higher doses are required. As the UV-C light with a shorter wavelength finds it difficult to penetrate longer distance through water, the visible light with a longer wavelength can easily pass through the water, giving rise to growth of algae. To maintain the UV dose to treat water effectively, a UV chamber must be designed to prevent the passage of long-wavelength visible light out of the reactor preventing algae growth and thereby maintaining the UV transmittance (UVT) values within the desired limit.

Innovative segregation of waste through a mechanized model: The mechanized segregation system can be developed for segregation of both live and dead wastes into different segments. A mechanized segregation unit of capacity 50 kg/h is developed as shown in Figure AII.3. Figure AII.4 shows the mechanized segregation unit for dead waste (capacity: 100 kg/h).

Disposal of plastic waste through pyrolysis: Pyrolysis is the thermal degradation of waste in the absence of air to generate gas often termed "syngas", pyrolysis oil and solid (char, mainly ash and carbon). The pyrolysis oil is being termed as "petro alternate fuel" (PAF), which can be used in industrial

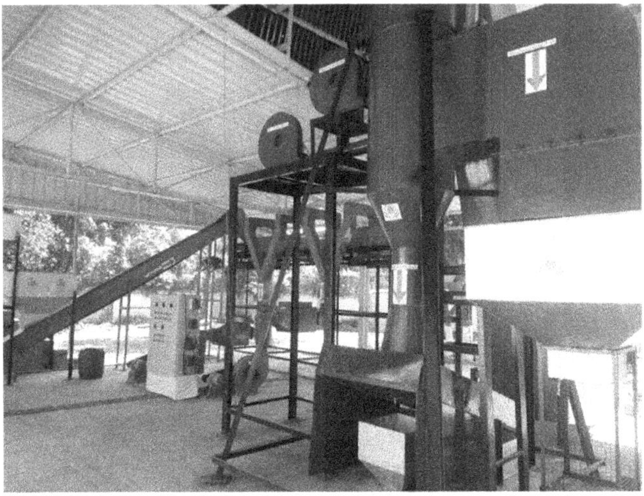

Figure AII.3 The mechanized segregation unit for live waste (capacity: 50 kg/h).

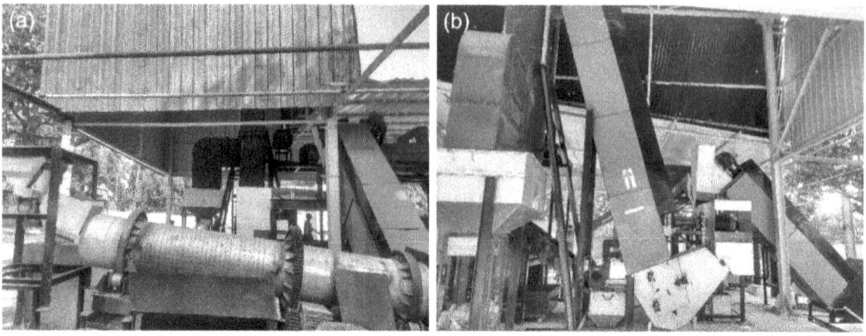

Figure AII.4 The mechanized segregation unit for dead waste (capacity: 100 kg/h).

Table AII.1 Major components of the polymer waste pyrolysis plant

Reactor	The reactor consists of a reaction vessel and a furnace which is insulated on the outside with ceramic wool and cladded. The reactor vessel is fed with raw material and catalyst mixed in a certain proportion. The furnace is heated so that the temperature inside the reactor is in a temperature range where catalytic decomposition takes place depending on various feedstocks. The heating system consists of an oil purification unit, an oil pumping unit and monoblock burners for oil and gas. The reactor also has the provision for nitrogen purging to create an inert environment to allow the process to happen in the absence of oxygen.
Gas receiver	The syngas from the catalytic degradation comes out of the reactor and is cleaned using a receiver where the heavier carbon particles and long chain hydrocarbons condense and flow back to the reactor and the lighter fraction is taken to the multilayer catalytic tower. The syngas velocity also decreases in the cyclone due to which the gas gets more residence time in the catalytic tower and subsequent line.
Catalytic tower	The catalytic tower is used to purify the syngas using catalysts in the vapor phase. Unwanted components like H_2S, SO_X, NO_X, etc. can be removed using appropriate catalysts, if required.
Condenser	Shell and tube condensers are used to cool the syngas from the reactor to liquid petro alternate fuel.
Anti-flashback device	The uncondensed clean gas is then passed through a tank that is partially filled with water. The gas bubbles out to the next line of components. The water ensures that the gas that bubbles out cannot go back to the previous line of components.
Scrubber	The gas and oil after getting fired in the furnace is cleaned by passing it through a wet alkali packed bed scrubber. The flue gas is cleaned, cooled and filtered to remove the particulate matter from the flue gas.
Chimney	The cooled flue gas is vented to the atmosphere through the chimney.
Flaring system	It is dangerous to vent exhaust gas (C1 to C4) without any safety measures. In this process, it is transferred first through the safety device and then burned in a burner or a flare system.
	Different heating mechanisms like solid fuel fired (briquette based), liquid fuel fired (diesel based) or gaseous fuel fired (biogas based) have been developed to compare the performance of the process in terms of energy efficiency. Also, the effect of the heating rate on product yield is studied.

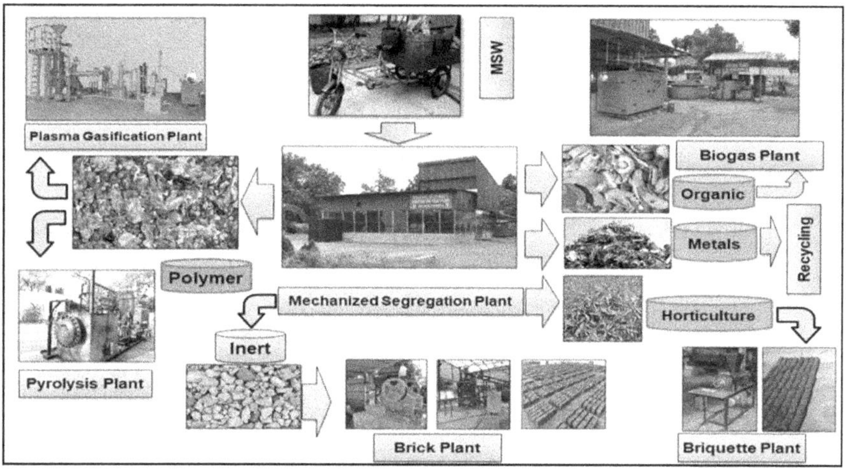

Figure AII.5 Cyclical decentralized solid waste disposal system.

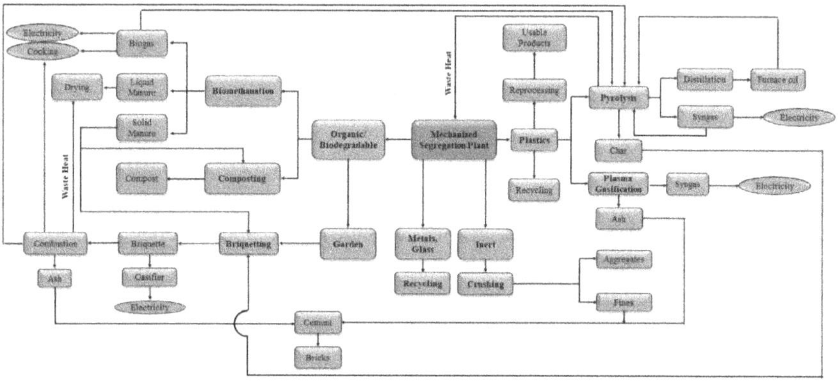

Figure AII.6 Mechanized segregation process flow chart.

boilers, generators or can be further refined into diesel. Table AII.1 shows the major components of the polymer waste pyrolysis plant.

Integrated municipal solid waste (MSW) management pilot plant: Day-to-day generated waste can be processed and colonies can be transformed into "Zero Waste Colony". This was experimented at a CSIR-CMERI colony. No waste has been discarded from the colony since January 2018. Figure AII.5 represents the developed cyclical decentralized solid waste disposal system, and the process flow chart of the mechanized segregation plant is given in Figure AII.6.

Figure AII.6 indicates inert waste, which are often construction debris that occupy valuable land resources coupled with soil and water pollution. Now through technological innovation, the construction debris can be

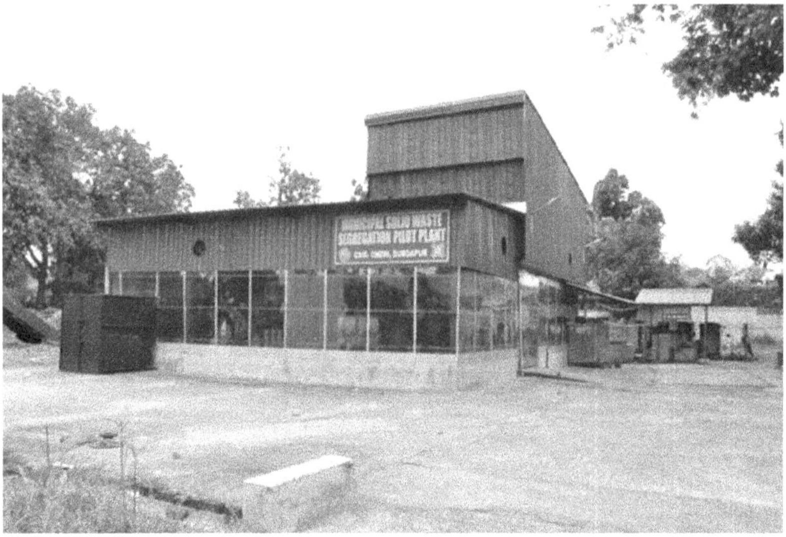

Figure AII.7 Developed *i*-MSWDS at CSIR-CMERI.

converted to bricks to construct parking spaces, partition wall, etc. The construction and demolition (C&D) debris is crushed in a jaw crusher and passed through a trommel to segregate crushed debris into different sizes. The fines (less than 5 mm) are mixed with cement and water in appropriate proportion and filled in the mold cavity of a hydraulic press to compact the mixture into proper brick shape. The bricks are cured to achieve the desired strength in the range of 15 –20 MPa. Finally, the physical properties of cured bricks are tested. Approved bricks can replace well-burnt red bricks. The oversized (5–20 mm) crushed materials may be used as aggregates in plain cement concrete (PCC) road making. When compared with conventional concrete as per the Central Public Works Department Delhi Schedule of Rate (CPWD DSR), the cost of C&D concrete is just 43% of conventional concrete.

Urban local bodies (ULBs), which are more popularly known as the municipal corporations or councils, are vetted with the responsibility for solid waste management in towns and cities. There is a possibility to improve financial management as a major chunk of fund is allocated for the transportation of waste materials from vats/bins to landfill sites and relatively little amounts are left for the most important steps – processing and recovery. To concur such situations the *i*ntegrated Municipal Solid Waste Disposal System (*i*-MSWDS) can be innovated by installing self-sufficient hybrid renewable energy systems based on solar photovoltaic (SPV) and biogas generators (Figure AII.7). Rooftop solar installation of 15 kWp capacity along with a 15 kVA biogas generator is sufficient to support the energy

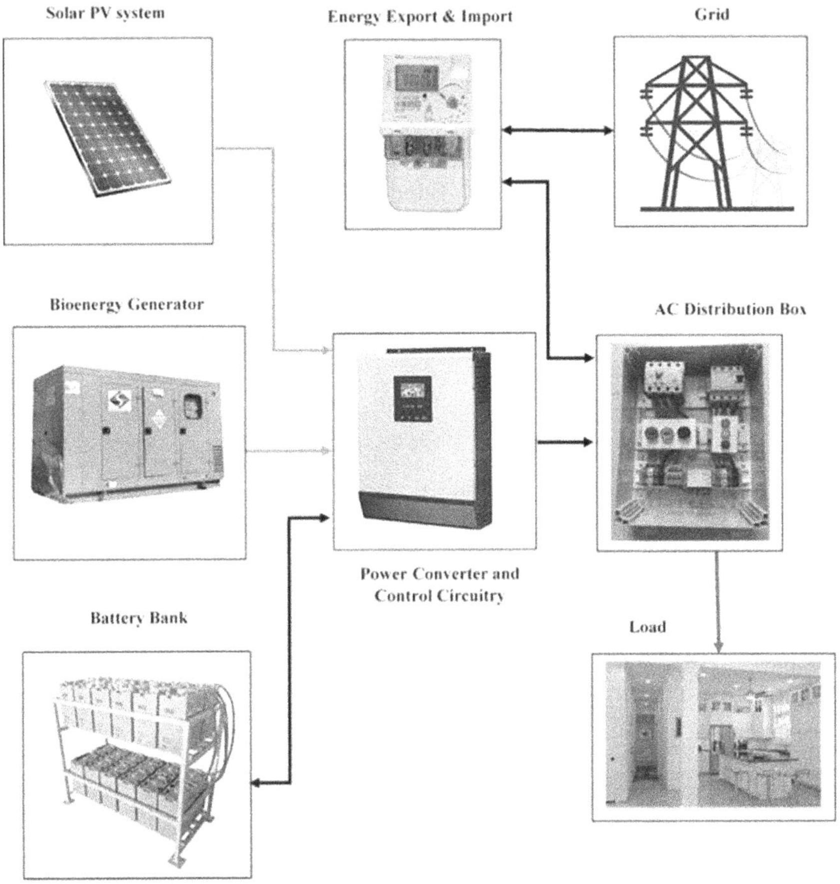

Figure AII.8 Schematic of the hybrid renewable energy system.

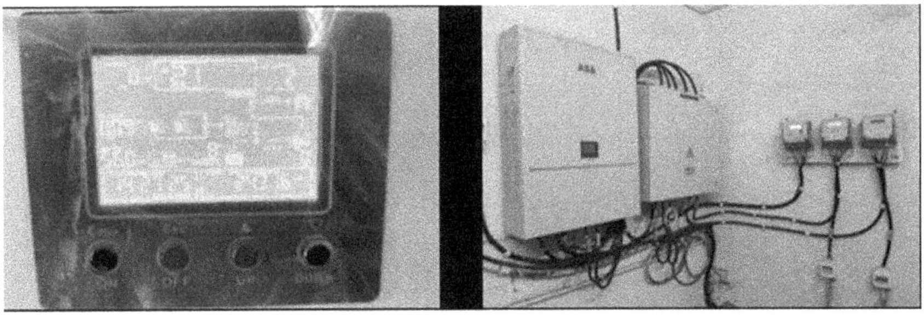

Figure AII.9 Electric connections and Digital display of the hybrid renewable energy system.

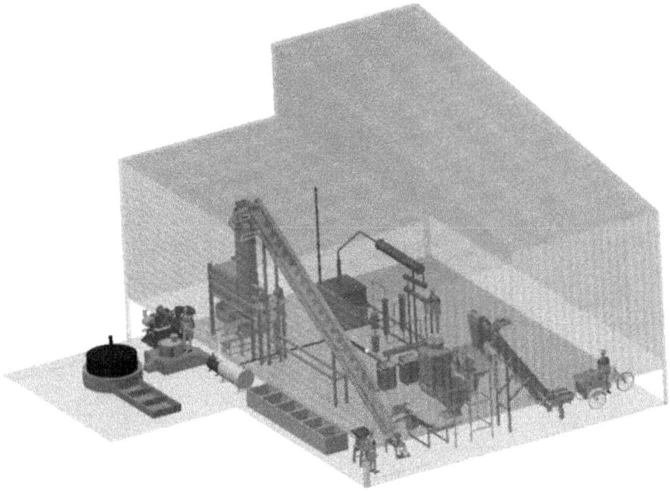

Figure AII.10 The hybrid renewable energy system for energy sustainability of the *inte*grated municipal solid waste disposal system (*i*-MSWDS).

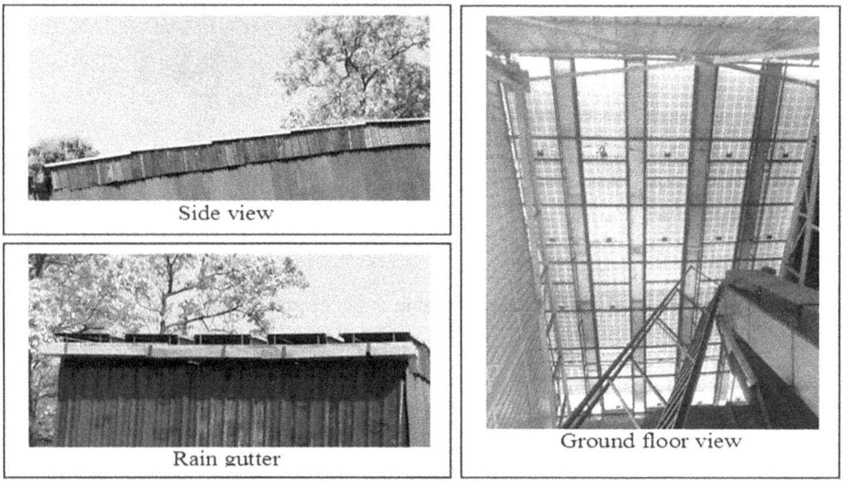

Figure AII.11 Rooftop solar installation in the *integrated municipal solid waste disposal* pilot plant at CMERI Colony.

requirement of a segregation pilot plant, plastic waste pyrolysis plant, biogas plant and briquette plant of 1 TPD. The provision of energy export–import facility is an added advantage since the extra energy produced by the hybrid system is fed to the electricity grid. The pyrolysis plant requires heat for its operation in addition to electricity and in order to make it self-sustainable. The generated pyrolysis oil is utilized for furnace heating after filtration and distillation. Additional supply of heat required to complete the process is obtained from combustion of biogas generated from biogas plants and the regenerated syngas making the process self-sustainable. The exhaust gas of combustion is passed through a recuperative air heater where the air is preheated to a suitable temperature. The preheated air is passed in the hot air conveying system of the segregation plant for reduction in the moisture content of the solid waste without utilizing any additional energy. The developed system is aimed toward reduction in the overall running expenditure of the plant by making it self-sustainable in terms of energy. The schematic of the hybrid renewable energy system is shown in Figures AII.8 and AII.9 and the hybrid renewable energy system for sustainability of the *i*ntegrated municipal solid waste disposal system (*i*-MSWDS) is shown in Figure AII.10. The rooftop solar installation in the *i*ntegrated municipal solid waste disposal pilot plant is shown in Figure AII.11.

BIBLIOGRAPHY

1. R.P. Bansal, and M. Goyal. *Activated Carbon Adsorption.* CRC Press, Taylor & Francis Group, Boca Raton, FL, 2005.
2. Ferhan Çeçen, and Özgür Aktaş. *Water and Wastewater Treatment: Historical Perspective of Activated Carbon Adsorption and its Integration with Biological Processes.* Wiley-VCH, Hoboken, NJ, 2011.
3. M.A. Giles, and R. Danell. Water dechlorination by activated carbon, ultraviolet radiation and sodium sulphite: a comparison of treatment systems suitable for fish culture. *Water Research*, 17:667–676, 1983.
4. Henze, M. *Biological Wastewater Treatment: Principles, Modelling and Design*, 2008th ed., vol. 96. IWA Publishing, London, UK, 2008.

Annexure III

Pneumatic precision planter for vegetables: Vegetables constitute about a 50% share among all horticultural produce and occupy an important place in the farm sector. Mechanization of these crops can increase efficiency and cost-effectiveness. Compared to the traditional methods of transplanting the nursery-raised seedlings, vegetable seeds can be directly planted to the required plant population using pneumatic precision planters. For choosing a precision planter, design of proper metering mechanism (i.e., pneumatic, belt, finger pickup and horizontal/inclined plates with cells) is the most important task. The pneumatic mechanism employs suction pressure for seed singulation of small seeds. A multirow (3/4/6 rows as per the tractor HP) precision planter, having a viewing window (for checking the vacuum on the seed plate and proper singulation), is suitable for majority of vegetable seeds. Important features of this unit are:

- Simple adjustments like seed plate change, plant spacing, depth and vacuum can be undertaken by unskilled farmers.
- Terrain following furrow opener (due to a parallelogram linkage system) ensures uniform depth of planting and germination.
- Height of the drive wheels can be adjusted for bed planting, furrow planting and ridge planting. Pneumatic tires for improved transmission from ground and easy transportation [see ref. 2 of Chapter 4].

Inter-row rotary cultivator for wide-row crops: Weeding and associated intercultural operation (shallow tilling and earthing) is a very important farm activity which is costly, tedious, time-consuming and a drudgery to the farm workers. The rotary cultivator is a perfect choice for farmers to undertake the weeding and intercultural operation. The prototype of an inter-row cultivator is shown in Figure AIII.1. The operational requirement and design consideration are shown in Table AIII.1.

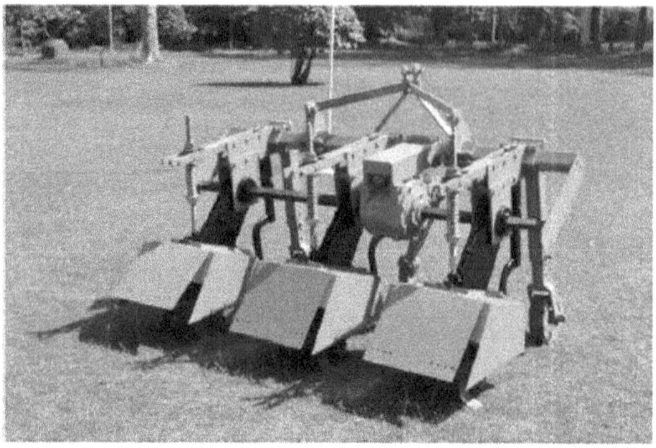

Figure AIII.1 Prototype of an inter-row cultivator.

Offset rotavator for orchards: To perform operations like tilling, inter-cultural rotavators may be utilized. To perform such operation under the canopies of the trees, there is a need of offsetting and side-shifting of the tilling unit to avoid damage to canopies. Important features that are desired from the machine are:

- Response time of the side-shifting mechanism must be low.
- Common tractor operators may be able to operate the offset rotavator.
- The rotavator must have provision of automatic hydraulic side-shift mechanism so that the damage to plants and also human fatigue can be minimized.
- The shield contours of the rotavator should be curved and shaped so as to avoid striking plants. Wheels can be deployed for a depth control system and should be placed in such a way that there is a considerable clearance from the end of the rotavator.
- The effective width of the rotavator can be about 2.13 m (7 ft) with a 0.91 m (3 ft) of achievable offset position. So, the performance of the machine is better in terms of field efficiency and field capacity.
- There should be provision of an offset lock in the rotavator because it is also equally important to cover the whole field area rather than concentrate on the area near trees only.

The rotavator is a tractor rear-mounted power takeoff (PTO)-operated hydraulic side-shift machine. The PTO of a tractor runs the hydraulic system and also the rotavator blades. Figure AIII.2 shows the front view of an offset rotavator. A schematic diagram of an offset rotavator is given in Figure AIII.3. The side-shift system is activated by a sensor fitted in the side of the rotary tiller and executed based on a hydraulic cylinder. The offset position of the rotavator can be

Table AIII.1 Operational requirement and design consideration of the inter-row cultivator

Ground clearance	Wide-row crops like sugarcane or cotton oversheds a height of 500–600 mm until completion of three weeding operations. The ground clearance of the tractor is to be 600 mm.
Depth of working, mm: 50–75	Most of the weeds get germinated from top 2 to 5 cm depth of the soil layer [see ref. 4 of Chapter 4]. However, we need a little more depth as we have little pulverization of soil to break up the capillaries and earthing up. Secondly, the pulverized soil will dry faster and thus re-emergence of weeds will reduce.
Bite length: 50–75 mm	Most of the rotary cultivators have a rotor speed of 300–350 rpm and a bite length of 60–70 mm. Also, the optimum length to be tilled in one bite should to be such that it should not leave any weeds in between, weeds get chopped and volume of soil being tilled is handled easily.
Working width: 500–550 mm	As most of the wide-row crops like sugarcane, cotton get cultivated at a row spacing of 675–900 mm. The covers of the weeding unit have a width of 560–580 mm and maintaining the remaining space for avoiding the injury to the crop.
Row spacing	As per agronomic package of practices, PAU, Ludhiana, 2011 [see ref. 5 of Chapter 4] • Sugarcane, mm: 675–900. • Cotton, mm: 675–900.
Selected design parameters for the machine developed are:	
Rotary blade rpm or gear ratio: 300–350, ~1.8. Bite length: 50–75 mm	
Cutting force of blades 250 N	It includes the total static and dynamic forces acting on the blade surface. Static force is dependent on the specific resistance of the soil. Dynamic force of rotary blades is dependent on energy required for throwing the soil layer, acceleration, and soil–metal friction force.
Shape of blade: trochoidal J shaped	Just scratching of the soil is needed along with weeds. However, maximum tillage depth up to 75 mm was considered as this will increase the pulverization of upper soil and will act as a capillary breaking and mulching activity which will suppress the next growth of weeds. Although C-shaped blades reduce the energy consumption, but to have greater shearing action perpendicular to the soil surface, L-shaped blade serves the purpose, but the energy consumption and surface area of the L-shaped blade is quite large. Hence, the optimum shape would be J-shape as it has a minimum surface area exposed to soil and its performance is also good. Hence, J-shaped blades were chosen. According to Sakai [see ref. 6 of Chapter 4], the coiling trouble of grass and straw to the rotary tillers occurred more easily on soft soils than on hard soil and generally weeding is done in tilled or soft soils. The grass-removing ability or blade would be better with the edge curve angle and thus the shape formed by the edge curve is called as trochoid.
Diameter of the rotor, 480–520 mm	Rotor diameters vary between 400 and 500 mm. Also, the blades used for the cultivator should have sufficient length to accommodate the trochoidal shape.

(*Continued*)

Table AIII.1 (Continued) Operational requirement and design consideration of the inter-row cultivator

Load on chain: 49.62 kN	Selected the chain as per BIS standards (1991) [see ref. 7 of Chapter 4] As the forces coming on the blade is ultimately carried forward to the chain drive, it comes to the conclusion (after calculations) of having this load and ultimately suggests us to select the higher breaking load chain.
Power requirement for rotary assembly: 7–8 kW	Calculated from the forces acting on blades and number of blades at a time in action.
Draft requirement for shovel: 1250–1350 N	Taking into account the unit draft of heavy soils and multiplying it with the cross-sectional area of soil slices.

Placement of gear box: Over the frame or on the transmission shaft.
Height of the PTO shaft from the ground: 650–700 (standard) mm
Standard 540 PTO RPM
Cat-II three-point linkages are preferred as majority of farmers opting for inter-row rotary weeders will have tractors of 50 hp or above.

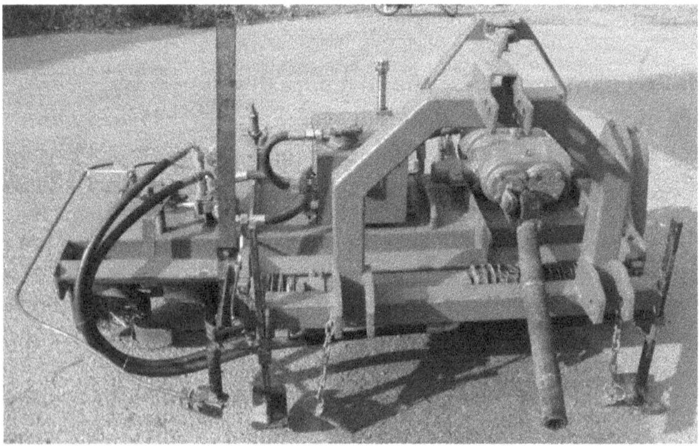

Figure AIII.2 Front view of an offset rotavator.

controlled by a hydraulic system which is operated by a sensor. The sensor touches the tree and pushes the hydraulic valve to side shift the machine automatically and bring it to a normal position behind the tractor. When the sensor passes a tree trunk and comes in free position, the rotavator moves in the offset position again. A double acting hydraulic cylinder is provided to adjust the offset position of the rotavator according to requirement of orchards. A curved shield is provided at the rear of the rotavator blades as a safety device.

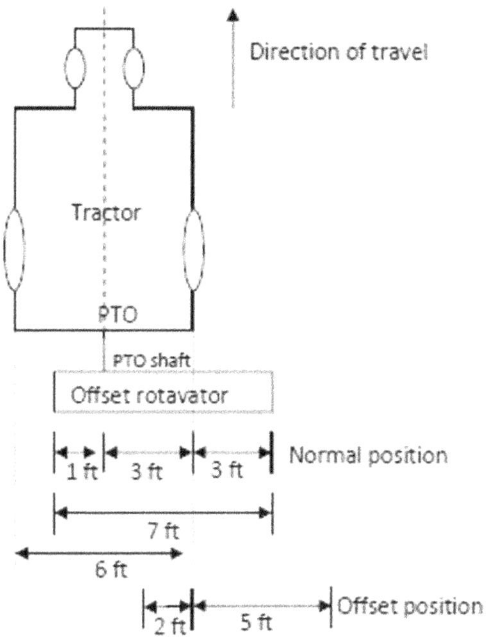

Figure AIII.3 Schematic diagram of an offset rotavator.

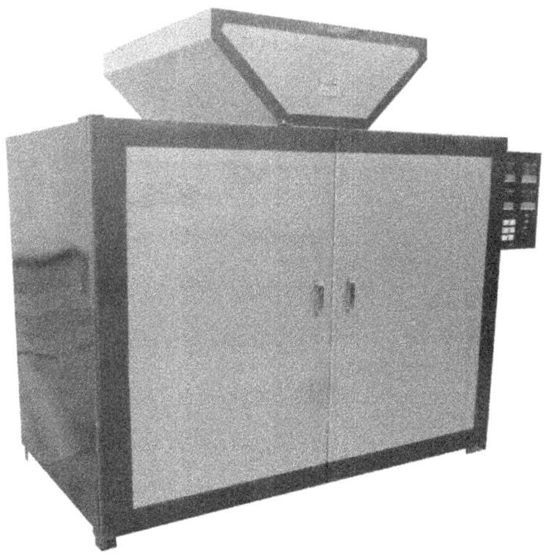

Figure AIII.4 Cabinet dryer.

***Ginger/turmeric processing technology:* cabinet dryer:** This dryer (shown in Figure AIII.4) is suitable for maintaining temperature in the range of 50–60°C for 40–50 kg/batch of perishable foods such as ginger, turmeric, potatoes, etc. A total electrical load of 15 kW is used to raise the temperature. The heat source is present at the bottom as well as at the middle which results in uniform drying of food placed on trays (made of SS 304; No. of trays: 16; Size of trays: 650 mm × 750 mm) kept inside the dryer.

***Ginger/turmeric processing technology:* slicing unit:** The slicing unit is shown in Figure AIII.5.

In this unit, washed gingers (or turmeric/potatoes) are loaded in the feeding hopper. The hopper is designed in such a manner that the ginger rhizomes are guided through the passage of the hopper to the cutter. The rotating cutter blades move over the ginger during rotation of the cutter and gingers are sheared off into flakes of desired thickness. The gingers are guided to the cutter blade one by one due to the jerk generated by the cutting action. Two cutters are mounted on the rotating back plate by mounting bolts providing enough peripheral space for the incoming ginger rhizomes. The thickness of the ginger flakes can be easily controlled by adjusting the gap between the cutter surface and the back plate. The sliced ginger flakes are discharged through a discharge chute. The technical specifications of the slicing unit are: gravity fed slicer; capacity of slicing: 50 Kg/h; the thickness

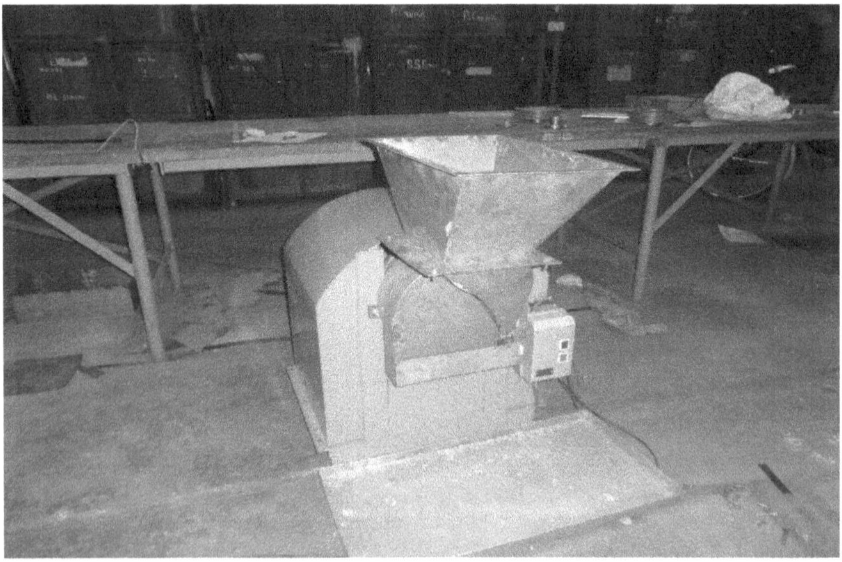

Figure AIII.5 Slicing unit.

of the slice may vary from 2 to 6 mm; motor 1.1 kW, 1000 rpm; ginger contacting material: SS-304.

Ginger/turmeric processing technology: **washing unit:** The developed rotating drum ginger washing machine consists of a feeding mechanism, cleaning with water jet spray in a rotating drum and discharging mechanism as shown in Figure AIII.6.

The raw ginger (or turmeric/potatoes) collected from the field is fed to the hopper which has a controllable discharge gate. The ginger is discharged to a vibrating tray at a controlled discharge rate at the outlet of the hopper. The vibrating tray mounted on four helical springs is vibrated by a vibrating electric motor. The vibrating tray gradually feeds gingers to the rotating drum. The vibration of the feed tray enhances the capacity of the washing unit. Using the perforated tray in the vibrating feeder, some soil material is screened out before feeding to the rotating drum. The rotating drum is perforated and powered by the drive arrangements consisting of electric motors, gear boxes, girth gears and pinions. The girth gear, pinion, supporting rim have been made with cast steel with case hardening. The drum rotates slowly at a rotational speed of about 5 rpm. The rotational speed of the drum has been selected in such a way to protect ginger rhizomes from wearing of external surfaces due to rubbing with the drum's internal surface. The drum has internal longitudinal fins along the length at a circumferential spacing. The drum is slightly inclined toward the discharge ends. As the drum rotates, the ginger inside it sweeps circumferentially and also moves toward the discharge end due to the combined effect of rotation and inclination of the drum. Water

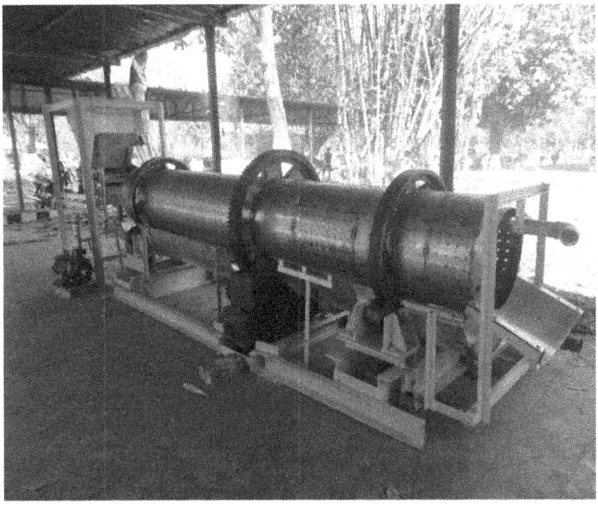

Figure AIII.6 Washing unit.

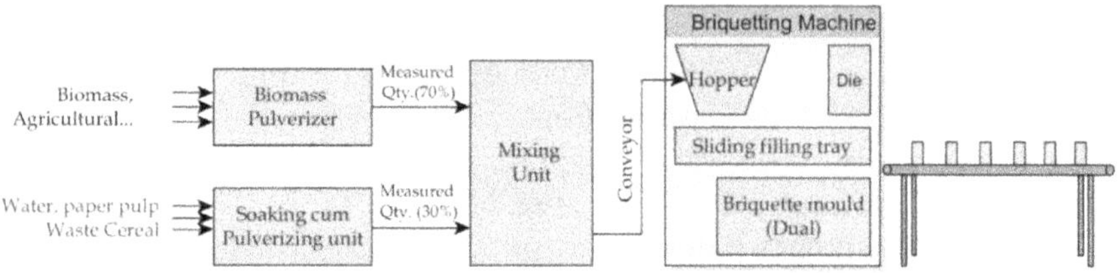

Figure AIII.7 Flow chart of the biomass briquetting process.

is sprinkled through a set of nozzles connected to the header pipe and pressurized water is supplied by a centrifugal pump. The used water can be recycled passing through a settling tank and after filtration. The gingers are cleaned by the water jets during its movement from the feed end to the discharge end. The cleaned ginger rhizomes are discharged through the discharge chute. All the components can be easily dismantled and reassembled which ensures for ease of transportation. The height of the ginger washing unit especially at the feed end is kept within the human reach for ease of operation. Technical specifications of the units are: duty: continuous type; capacity of washing: 250 kg/h; drum diameter: 500 mm; drum length: 3500 mm; motor: 2.2 kW, 1450 rpm; drum speed: 5–6 rpm; vibrating feeder; ginger contacting material: SS-304 ASTM A 240.

Automatic biomass briquetting plant: A multi-feedstock automatic briquetting machine can be developed to produce briquettes offsite from agro wastes like paddy straw, dry leaves, rice husk, grass, sawdust, etc. In general, the feedstocks (straw, dry leaves, grass, etc.) are chopped into a size of 2 mm to 1.5 cm in a shredder. A binder is prepared by mixing starch or paper pulp with water. Thereafter, both the feedstock and the binder come to a pan mixer where they are thoroughly mixed and transferred to the main briquetting machine hopper through a vertical screw conveyor. From the hopper, the raw material flows down to a feeding box through gravity and through a preprogrammed process (through PLC) briquettes are produced and transferred through a roller conveyor. Thereafter, the briquettes can be dried in a conventional/solar dryer up to a moisture content of less than 5% for final use for cooking purposes or for generation of heat in boilers and furnaces.

The briquettes produced through the optimized process have been found to have a calorific value of 3000–6000 kCal/kg, a prolonged burning time of 20–60 minutes, low ash content and fixed carbon (5% each), less chloride (0.02%) and sulfur content (0.3%) [see ref. 8 of Chapter 4]. Figure AIII.7 depicts the flow chart of the biomass briquetting process. A write-up on the

Table AIII.2 Contribution made vis-à-vis comparative international position in biomass briquetting

Sl. no.	*Open burning of leaves/grass/rice straw*	*Burning of Briquettes made from dry leaves/ grass/rice straw*
1.	Energy is wasted into nature.	Energy is utilized for heat generation.
2.	Space requirement for burning is more.	Due to densification, size of burning space is far less.
3.	Calorific value generated is less per unit volume.	Calorific value generated is higher due to densification and addition of binders.
4	Smoke produced is high.	Smoke produced is less.

contribution made vis-à-vis comparative international position is given in Table AIII.2.

Annexure IV

Machining: Machining requires a cutting tool to remove the excess material by shearing action. Three main machining operations: turning, milling and drilling are described in this section.

- **Turning:** Lathe machine is a versatile available machine in almost every workshop. Turning operation performed on the lathe machine subtracts the material (Figure AIV.1) from the surface of a rotating cylindrical workpiece to reduce the diameter to the desirable dimension having a smooth metallic finish. Following are some of the steps to be followed to avoid any mistake during turning operation:
  - After loading the workpiece on the chuck/faceplate, it is advisable to rotate the workpiece manually to ensure no physical contact of the workpiece with any part of the lathe.
  - Position the cutting tool away from the chuck or lathe dog before starting the machine, otherwise the tool may strike with them during rotation.
  - Before starting the lathe, ensure that the component is properly clamped in the chuck. Similarly, secured clamping of the tail stock and tool rests is to be confirmed.
  - Prior to starting the lathe, ensure that the long small-diameter workpiece is also supported from the tail stock center.
  - The operator must ensure the proper direction and speed of the carriage or cross feed to avoid any kind of fouling before engaging the automatic feed.
  - Ensure no excess pieces of stock, tools and bits are present on the machine bed.
  - Ensure guarding of all the belts and pulleys before starting the machine.

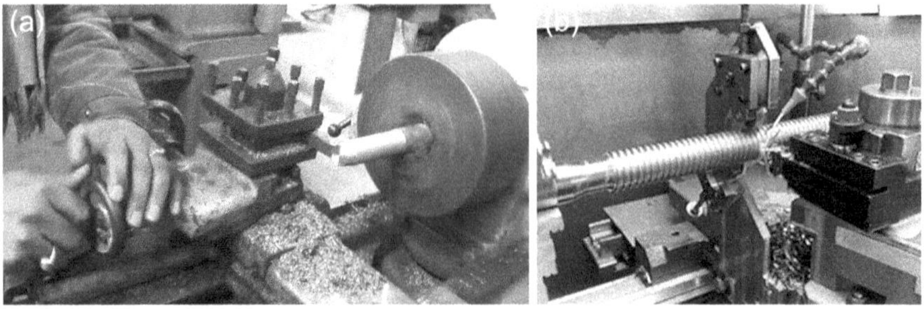

Figure AIV.1 Turning operation on the lathe machine.

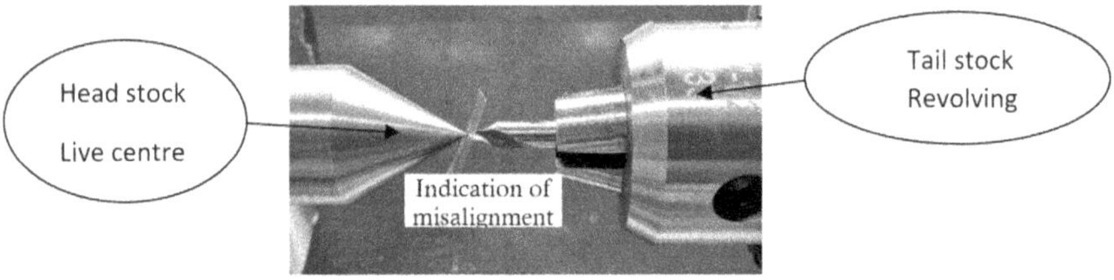

Figure AIV.2 Checking alignment of headstock and tailstock centers.

- In case of any odd (unusual) noise or excessive vibration observed from the machine, the machine should be stopped immediately for taking suitable corrective action by maintenance personnel.
- To execute threading operation (as shown in Figure AIV.1) on lathe machines, special care must be taken to set the speed to about one quarter of the speed used for turning. Set the quick-change gearbox for the required pitch in threads. Set the compound rest at right angle and choose appropriate thread tool bit.
- Lathe machines are subjected to wear and aging. To enhance the serviceability of the lathe machine, regular inspection (*i.e., coolant levels, lubricant levels for a centralized and circulating lubrication system*) and maintenance (*i.e., cleaning loose chips/debris/dust, cleaning oil strainers, timely lubrication of prescribed parts*) of the lathe machine is very important. The regular maintenance also ensures good surface roughness and dimension tolerances of the workpiece.
- To minimize the tool wear and avoid the damage of the workpiece, ensure appropriate center height setting of tools. One way to properly set the tool is to crosscheck the tailstock's alignment as shown below in Figure AIV.2, wherein the alignment between the headstock live center and tailstock revolving center is being crosschecked and needs to be properly aligned.

– Use tailstock support for longer, thinner and/or heavier workpiece. The dead center in the tailstock allows a workpiece to spin freely while still being supported. A workpiece mounted in this way is said to be turned “between centers”. Besides that, the tailstock can be used to mount a drill bit or other tools too.

- **Milling:** It is a process performed with a rotating cutter to subtract the material from the rectangular/square bar. Unlike lathe, where the workpiece is rotated against the tool, a milling cutter spins against the workpiece. Due to such relative motion between the tool and the workpiece, a variety of operations, such as shown in Figure AIV.3, can be performed on a milling machine. Various types of milling cutters to be used on both conventional type horizontal and vertical milling machines including tools required for pocket machining and 3D surface machining on computer numerical control (CNC) machines are shown in Figure AIV.4. Following are some of the steps to be followed to avoid any mistake during milling operation:
  – Pay proper attention to holding the workpiece on the machine table (either directly on the table or in the vice) to avoid physical displacement of the workpiece relative to the machine

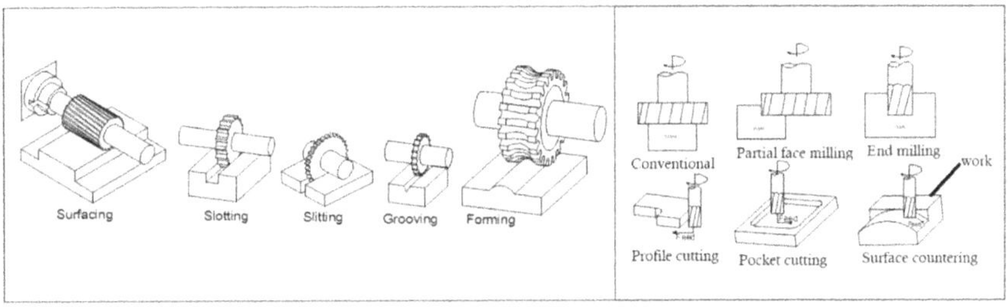

Figure AIV.3 Different milling operations and arrangements of cutter vs workpiece.

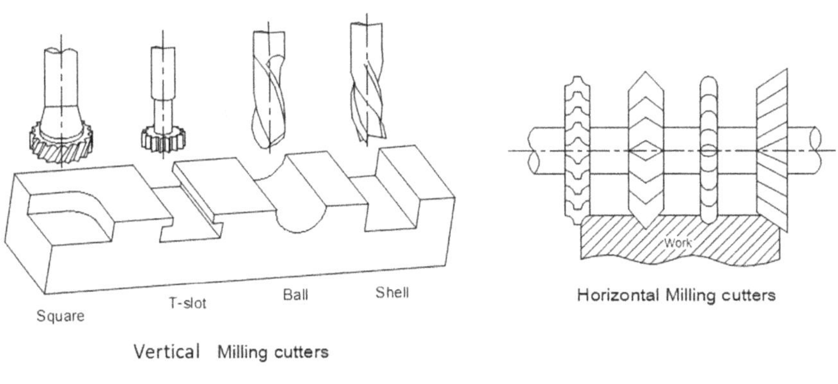

Figure AIV.4 Milling cutters and their axes of rotation.

table, otherwise damage to the cutter, machine, operator, etc. may occur. Usually workpieces are positioned in a vice above the vice jaws by putting parallel bars of the same height and proper size below the component. Heights of the parallel bars should be selected wisely to raise the component just enough to allow the required cut. While holding the workpiece on parallels, a soft hammer should be used to tap the top surface of the piece after the vice jaws have been tightened.

- There is a need to select appropriate cutting parameters such as "n: number of revolutions of the spindle in one minute"; "D_c: cutter diameter in millimeter"; "v_c: cutting speed in meters per minute $\left(v_c = \frac{\pi D_c n}{1000}\right)$"; "$f_f$: advancement of the work table during one revolution of the rotating cutter"; "v_f: speed at which the table advances against the rotating cutter in millimeters per minute ($v_f = f_f n$)"; "f_z: advancement of the work table during the rotational movement of the cutter between two cutting edges $\left(f_z = \frac{f_f}{z} = \frac{v_f}{z.n}\right)$". The cutting speed ($v_c$) is adjusted based on the type of component material, type and material of the cutting tool used and also based on the rigidity of the clamping. It is preferred to use the values of the cutting speed (v_c) and the cutter diameter (D_c) in the formula so that the rotational speed "n" of the spindle can be calculated in rotations/revolutions per minute (RPM). To calculate the axial feed rate (V_f) of the work table in millimeters per minute, the values of both feed (f_f) per revolution and number of cutter's revolutions (n) per minute are required. The value of feed per revolution is required to be checked against the manufacturer's guidelines.
- Appropriate tool setting (i.e., minimizing tool overhung, right tool speed and feed rate, type of tool and coolant) is essential to avoid the problem of chattering or vibration. The chatter or vibration can generate a loud and dissonant noise during milling, and unpleasant wavy marks are observed on the machined part by reducing the surface quality and also shortening the tool/machine life. This problem can be solved/reduced by giving proper skill development training. Figure AIV.5 shows the surfaces generated by milling with stable machining conditions and with unstable machining conditions.

- **Drilling:** Drilling is a very common cutting process to produce holes of circular cross-section in the solid material. It is important to understand that for every drilling operation, the first and foremost requirement is the need of indentation to be created by center

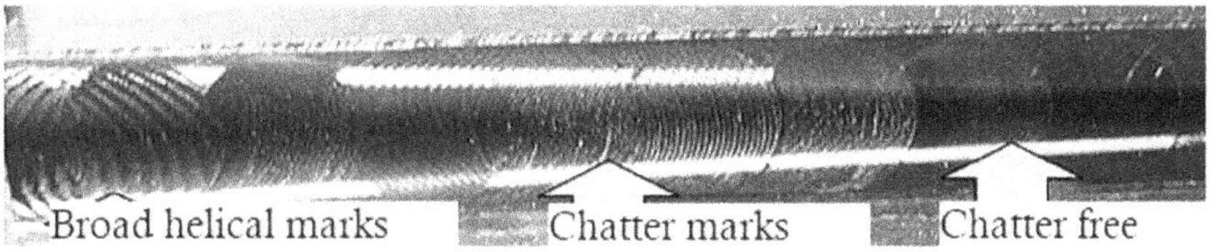

Figure AIV.5 Generated milled surfaces with (a) number of flutes and (b) optimized feed and speed conditions.

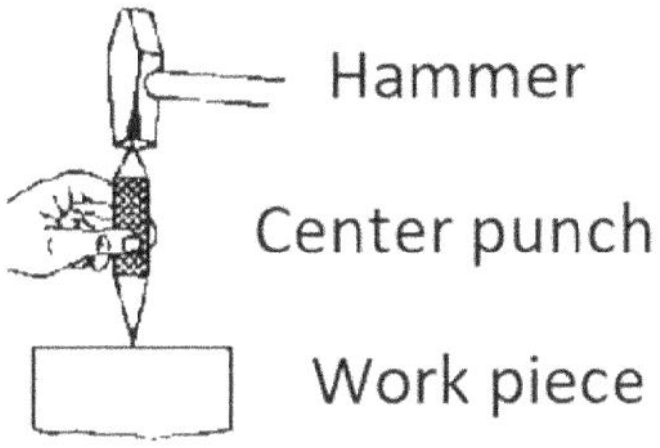

Figure AIV.6 Punch marking to create the center point.

punch/center drilling operation (shown in Figure AIV.6), which acts as a guide to generate appropriate holes; otherwise, if the drill is directly initiated on a flat surface, then the drill tip tends to run away from the center and causes the drill to advance in an angular direction and sometime causing the drill to break in the process. After drilling operation, the internal surface of the hole is relatively rough. Additional problem is sizing as the drilled hole becomes bigger than the drill size (i.e., a drill of 12 mm diameter makes a hole of approx. 12.125 mm). A drill with a flat end produces a flat surface and is used for making counterbores. Stepped drills are used to produce holes of different diameters by using a single tool. Pilot drills are used to produce little accurate holes by taking the guide of the previously drilled holes. Reamers are used to produce most accurate holes with proper surface finish and required hole size. Reaming operation is done after creating a hole by drilling operation with a size less than the reamer size by keeping suitable allowance for reaming operation. Figure AIV.7 provides illustration of the type of operations that can be done by a drill machine and the type of tools needed for carrying out those operations.

Similarly, gun drilling operation is used for producing straight and long bores/holes. Counter sinking operations are used to provide a chamfering on the edges of the drilled holes by using a cutter with a shape to provide the required angle of the chamfer on the edge of the holes.

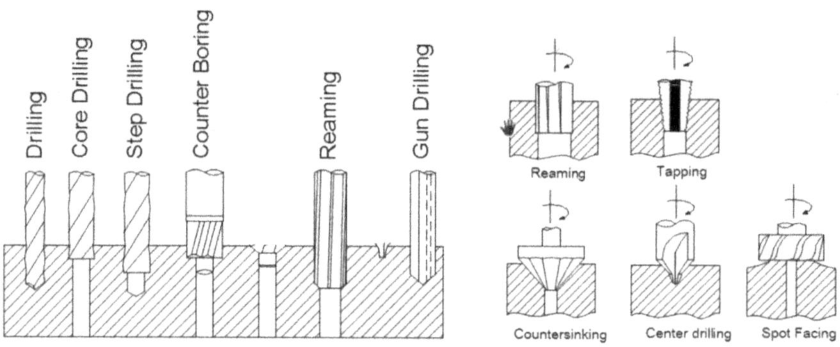

Figure AIV.7 Different types of drilling operations and respective tool shapes.

Finally tapping operation is used to produce internal threads inside a drilled hole by using a tool called "tap" which has an external threaded surface to suit the thread shape to be produced inside the hole.

Most of the small and medium enterprises (SMEs) choose high-speed steel (HSS) drills for drilling operations on a radial drilling machine. Based on the diameter of the drill being used speed has to be selected by using the available combination of the gear mechanism. It is very important to convey the importance of selecting proper speed and feed by following the charts provided by the machine manufacturer. Table IV.1 gives drilling speeds for different materials and Figure AIV.8 provides the formula for calculating speed and feed for drilling operation. Similar to milling operations, cutting parameters, for drilling operation too, are calculated by using the formula as provided in Figure AIV.8. The first part of the formula explains how to calculate the cutting speed (v_c) by putting the suitable values of the cutter diameter in millimeters and spindle speed in revolutions per minute. The cutter diameter will be recorded after accurately measuring it by using either a vernier caliper or a micrometer screw gauge, whereas the spindle speed (n) is selected based on the type of component material and tool material by referring to the cutting tool manufacturer's guidelines and the value of (n) depends upon the maximum speed available in the machine spindle. The second part of the formula explains how to calculate the spindle speed (RPM) by putting the suitable values of the cutter diameter in millimeters and cutting speed in meters per minute. The cutting speed v_c is selected based on the type of component material and tool material by referring to the cutting tool manufacturer's guidelines. The third part of the formula explains how to calculate the cutting feed in millimeters per minute by putting the values of spindle speed (n) and feed rate per revolution (f) in millimeters per revolution. Similarly, the fourth part of the formula helps to calculate the feed rate per revolution

Table IV.1 Drilling speeds for different materials with high-speed steel drills [need to use the table provided by drill machine OEM]

Drill Dia. mm	Drill Speed rpm			
	Steel	Cast Iron	Iron	Alum. & Copper
3	1580	2580	2580	2580
4	1350	2180	2180	2580
5	1290	1580	1580	2580
6	830	1350	1350	2580
7	830	1290	1290	2580
8	830	1290	1290	2580
9	540	830	830	2180
10	500	830	830	2180
11	500	830	830	1580
12	420	830	540	1580
13	420	540	540	1350
14	420	540	500	1350
16	320	500	500	1290
18	320	420	420	1290
20	280	320	320	1290
22	210	320	280	830
25	210	280	210	830

1. Calculation of cutting speed

$$VC = \frac{\pi \times DC \times n}{1000}$$

2. Calculation of rotational speed

$$n = \frac{1000 \times VC}{\pi \times DC}$$

3. Calculation of feed speed per minute

$$Vf = n \times f$$

4. Calculation of feed rate per revolution

$$f = \frac{Vf}{n}$$

5. Calculation of drilling time

$$T = \frac{H}{Vf}$$

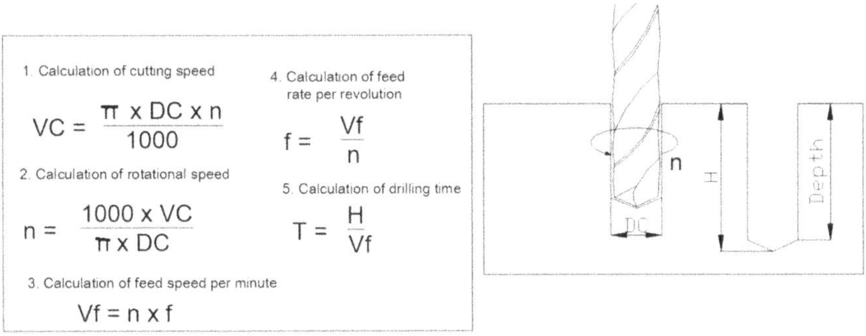

Figure AIV.8 Formulas for calculation of cutting parameters in drilling operations.

by putting the values of feed rate per minute and spindle speed (n) in the formula. And finally, the fifth part of the formula explains how to calculate time required for completion of a drilling operation by dividing the length of the drilling in millimeters with feed rate in millimeters per minute (V_f).

New operators must be trained to know that drill should always rotate in the correct direction otherwise drills start rubbing instead

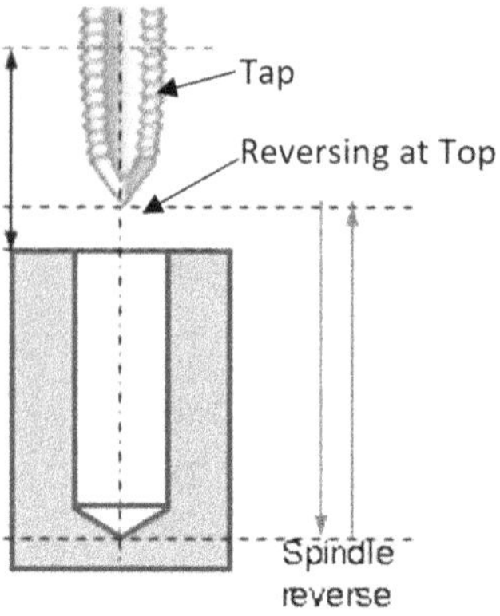

It can be observed in the side figure that the tap starts in one direction at the top and it reverses its direction of rotation after reaching the bottom. Similarly, it reaches back to top point in the same direction and again reverses its direction after reaching the top position.

Figure AIV.9 Reversing of the spindle rotation direction during tapping operation.

of cutting by generating enormous heat, which damages both the drill and the component. It is also to be taught to new operators that in some cases drills are run in the reverse direction (if the drill is left-handed). Even during tapping operation, direction of rotation has to be reversed during the retraction of tap from the hole as explained in Figure AIV.9. It is necessary to use a coolant during drilling operation as it plays three important roles: removing generated heat, cleaning the work surface and the drill and maintaining better surfaces. Very often SMEs commit mistakes by using plain water as a coolant which can remove the heat but increases chances of rusting on both the component and the machine tool. In addition, water alone cannot remove the metal residues which get deposited on the flutes during drilling operation. Cleaning the deposits after every use is important to ensure that the drill can perform better and provide better service life.

Welding positions: The position of a welded joint refers to its relationship with the horizontal plane. Different types of positions are horizontal filet welding (img.1), vertical filet welding (img.2), overhead filet welding (img.3), flat butt welding (img.4), overhead butt welding (img.5), vertical butt welding (img.6), as mentioned in Figure AIV.10.

WELDING TECHNIQUES

- **Leftward or forward welding:** In this welding progresses in the forward direction, i.e., from right to left. The blowpipe is held firmly at an angle of 60°–70° with the plane of the weld and moved forward in such a way that flame points in the direction of travel. The filler rod stays between 30° and 40°.

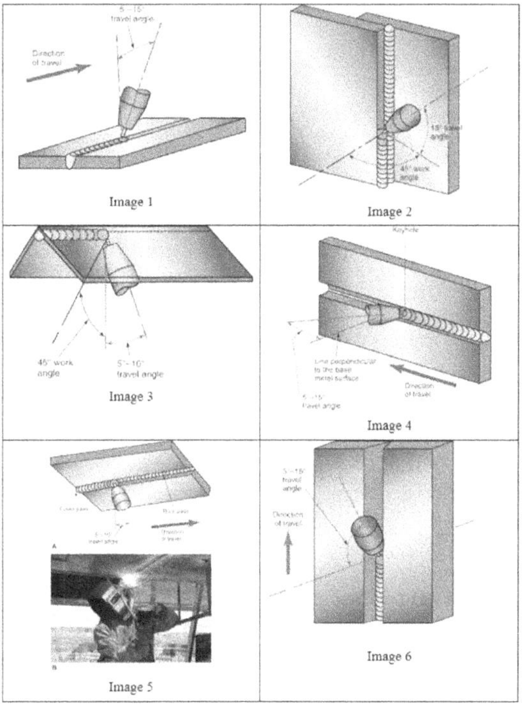

Figure AIV.10 Welding positions.

- **Rightward or backward welding:** This method is employed for welding of thicker plates. The blowpipe and the filler rod are held at an inclination with the plane of weld at 40°–50° and 30°–40°, respectively.

Aluminum casting: Al–Mg alloy casting requires appropriate drying of mold skin, as magnesium reacts with the water vapor and may cause pinholes and microporosity. If the metal is poured quickly after closing the mold, skin drying is enough. Delayed casting requires complete drying of the mold; otherwise, the moisture from the inside of the mold will diffuse to the outer plate of the dry mold, causing defects in the cast parts. Good results are obtained with molds coated with hexachloroethane or hexachlorobenzene and sand molds with boric acid.

A non-pressurized gate (inlet area ≥ runner area > sprue area) as shown in Figure AIV.11 should be used to allow the mold to be quickly filled with negligible turbulence. Since aluminum alloys have a higher coefficient of thermal expansion, it expands further during melting and the component contracts heavily during solidification. Therefore, large size risers should be used to compensate for the shrinkage. The runners should also have

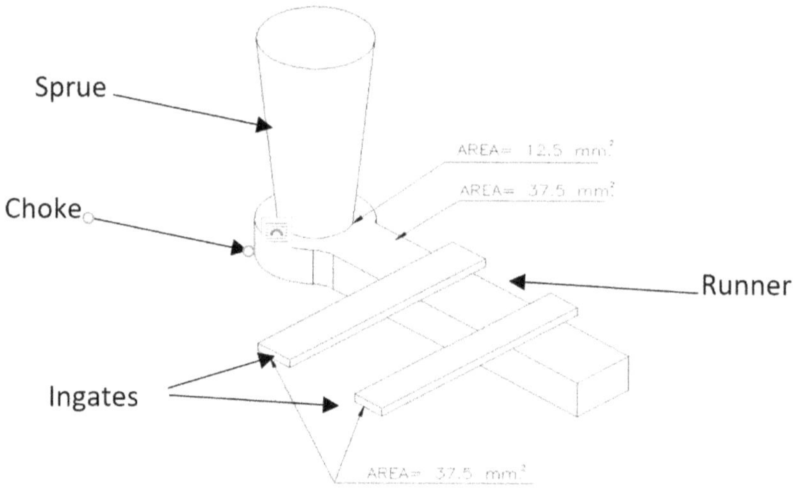

Figure AIV.11 The non-pressurized gating system.

sufficient extension to avoid air entrapment in the casting. Also, the streamlining of molten metal flow is very beneficial for complete filling of the mold.

- **Charging:** The aluminum alloy ingots should be cleaned properly before charging. Avoid machined aluminum chips as they may contain lubricants. During charging of aluminum alloy, the low melting point alloying elements like Zn and Mg should be added in elemental form with a phosphorizer for deoxidation and capturing hydrogen gas and other elements should be used in the form of hardener alloys.
- **Deoxidation and degassing:** Flux is used to combine with oxides on the surface of the melt. This generates viscous slag and protects the base metal from additional oxidative attacks. Therefore, to homogenize, the melt must be agitated from bottom to top without excessively destroying the surface. Flux is essential if the amount of cast scrap in the batch is too large. Foundries operating high-speed crucible furnaces rarely use flux to minimize the risk of contamination. Proper degassing eliminates the possibility of defects due to gaseous elements. For melting aluminum alloys, C_2Cl_6 (hexachloroethane) tablets are preferred over chlorine gas. Gas purging is more effective than adding salt to degassing because chloride salts take longer to decompose, release chlorine and remove hydrogen. If not properly dried, it may introduce gas instead of removing it. C_2Cl_6 not only degases the melt but also refines the grain (heterogeneous nucleation). Currently, it is common to use SF_6 (sulfur hexafluoride) as the carrier

gas. It is better than the previous method because it does not harm the environment.

- In the gas purge process, nitrogen/argon is typically introduced into the melt via a graphite rod, porous plug or high-speed rotor. Theoretically, until the thermochemical equilibrium is reached. The residence time of bubbles in the melt is usually in the range of a few seconds and usually does not reach equilibrium.

Process of Dokra casting: This process is an ancient tradition of Asia, Africa and Pan-Pacific regions and is still followed in many regions of India, Bangladesh, Papua New Guinea and Benin of West Africa. An extensive study was conducted in different villages of Eastern India and the technique of manufacturing is as follows:

Stage 1: A mixture of clay, rice husk and sand (40–60 AFS No.) in the ratio of 4:1:1, with appropriate moisture, is required for making the clay core.

Stage 2: The formed core is dried under the sun and the top surface is given finishing touch.

Stage 3: After appropriate drying, waxing is done along with suitable runners and gates, made of the same wax. For coreless or solid castings, the process starts from this stage with making of the wax pattern as shown in Figure AIV.12.

Stage 4: To make hollow casting, 3–5 mm thick investment shells of clay and cow dung mixture is pasted over the wax pattern and then dried slowly. The clay used here is of fine clay type collected by artisans. Covering the investment shell, another backup layer of the clay-sand-rice husk aggregate of generous thickness (minimum

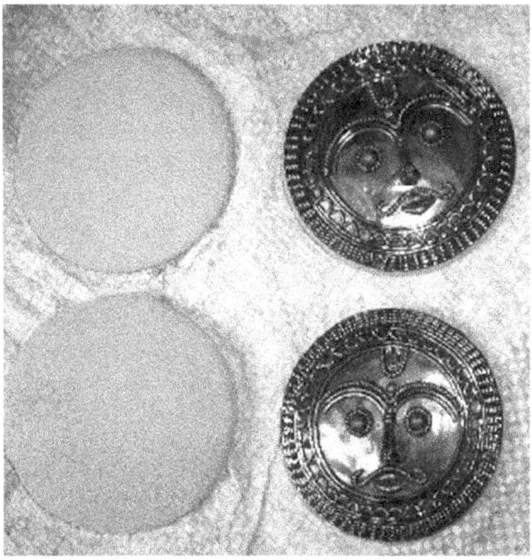

Figure AIV.12 The dried clay core (left) and the finished wax pattern.

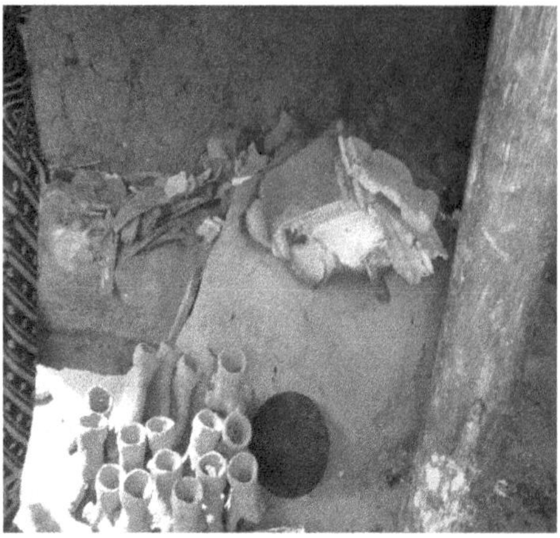

Figure AIV.13 Traditional Dokra casting in progress.

6 mm) is applied, with the making of a funnel at the gate, to hold the metal. Then, the whole of this mold is sun dried.

Stage 5: When the metal is separately melted for casting, then the investment mold is directly transferred to a pit furnace and gradually heated in coal fire for dewaxing and casting. But, in case, when the metal is melted within the integrated mold, the metal pieces are placed in the funnel of the mold. The funnel is then covered by a green clay cap. An opening is kept at the top of the funnel. Brass or bronze scraps generally are charged into the mold, eight to ten times the weight of the wax. More metal is melted than is necessary to have a continuous flow of liquid metal and avoid shrinkage due to volume contraction. The total mold is heated in a steam coal fire at around 1100°C for first dewaxing and then melting the solid metal into liquid.

Stage 6: Metal is melted in a graphite crucible (Figure AIV.13) on a coal-fired pit furnace and then the hot metal is poured without any interruption by the preheated dewaxed investment clay mold, like any other conventional casting process. When the casting cools, usual fettling, brushing and repairing by soldering (if any) are done. For finishing the casting surface, it is polished with soapnut/tamarind solution. After finishing, the casting (Figure AIV.14) becomes ready for shipment.

The problems and remedies related to Dokra casting: Problems or defects in Dokra casting can generally be divided into: (a) distortion, (b) poor surface finish, (c) fins, (d) rough surface, (e) porosity, (f) voids, (g) incomplete

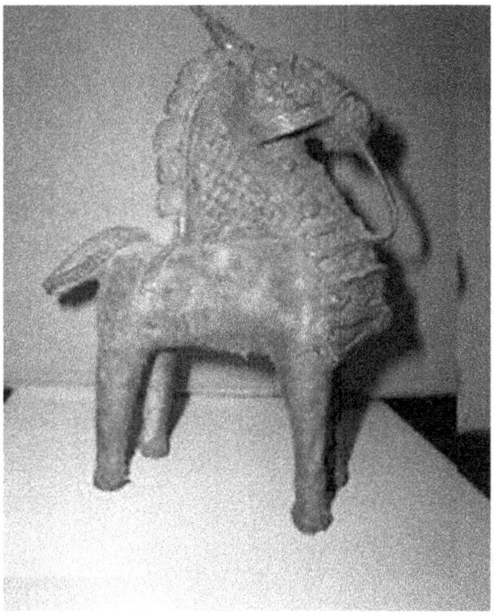

Figure AIV.14 A traditional Dokra casting.

filling and (h) low yield. These imperfections are of general nature and part of any metal casting process as well as Dokra casting process.

To improve these defects a low-cost and fuel-efficient furnace has been developed that can melt 8–12 kg of metal per batch and control the pouring temperature effectively. In addition to this, methoding (design of gating and risering system) of casting has been done using casting simulation software. By introducing proper methoding and melting practice, the quality of the castings can been improved and rejection of the casting can decreased.

Smart foundry: In this section, an overview of concept development for SMART FOUNDRY at CSIR-CMERI are discussed. The "SMART Foundry" is a complete advanced foundry for the casting of small aluminum components of up to 2 kg. The overall system footprint will fit inside a 12 ft × 12 ft size room. The system is composed of six major system components as mentioned below:

Simulation software: Two technical software, (1) for tooling and method design and (2) a computer fluid dynamics (CFD)-based multiphysics solver for casting process simulation, have been developed. The final optimized 3D component is then forwarded for 3D printing.

3D printer: This is being used for three-dimensional printing of patterns. From a 3D-computer-aided design (CAD) model of the pattern with all requisite allowances, the pattern is printed using acrylonitrile butadiene styrene (ABS) thermoplastics. After layer-by-layer printing, the pattern can also be treated by vapor polishing operation for achieving superior surface finish as per requirement. The required runner and risers are also printed with the pattern in this unit.

Automatic molding machine: This subsystem is used for the generation of sand molds using the pattern printed by a 3D printer. This subsystem consists of five components.

A. A sand container with an automated valve: for discharging the required quantity of sand, automatic resin, and hardener pumping systems are also there for feeding a controlled amount of mentioned ingredients for sand molding.
B. Sand mixer: This is equipped with a motorized blade for mixing sand, resin and hardener. The mixing speed and time can be controlled as per process requirements. After completion of mixing, there is an actuator-controlled gate for discharging the molding mass into the mold box.
C. Automatic mold box assembly: Actuator-controlled automatic mold box assembly enables opening and closing of the mold box for ease of extraction of mold. There is a provision in the match plate for providing some jolting action for evenly spreading of the molding mass.
D. Ramming station: On receiving sensor input after pouring sand into the mold box, the ramming station comes into position and exerts the required force for compaction through the actuator-controlled ramming plate.
E. Central controller: Equipped with a graphical user interface (GUI) for feeding process parameters, the central controller controls the subsystem operation.

Melting and pouring unit: After preparation of the mold, it is placed in this unit. It is equipped with a bottom pouring furnace that melts and pours the aluminum in the mold for casting of the component. There is a provision in the system for attachment units like vacuum/inert gas units and metal matrix composites.

Internet of things (IoT)-enabled smart features in SMART FOUNDRY: An architecture is designed for enabling the smart features in SMART FOUNDRY. A graphical user interface (GUI) is also developed for implementing IoT technology in the SMART FOUNDRY concept as shown in Figure AIV.15. It is designed and developed using three layers as given below:

- Hardware layer: Sensor and actuators, motor, microcontroller, etc.
- Server/internet layer: Communication devices like gateway/router, internet server, cloud platform, configuration of IP in server.
- End user/ application layer: Display interface devices like PC, mobile, etc.

Operation steps: In the system, sand needs to be mixed with a hardener, and ramming of sand filled in the mold is to be performed. The sand is

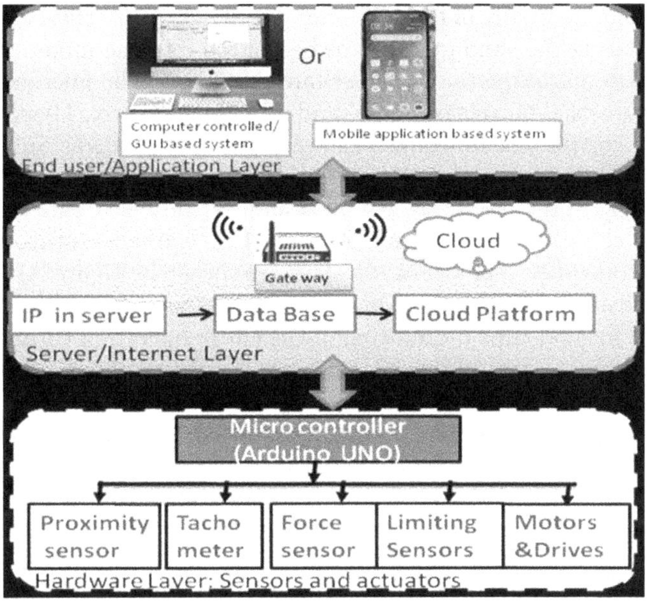

Figure AIV.15 IoT-enabled smart architecture design for SMART FOUNDRY.

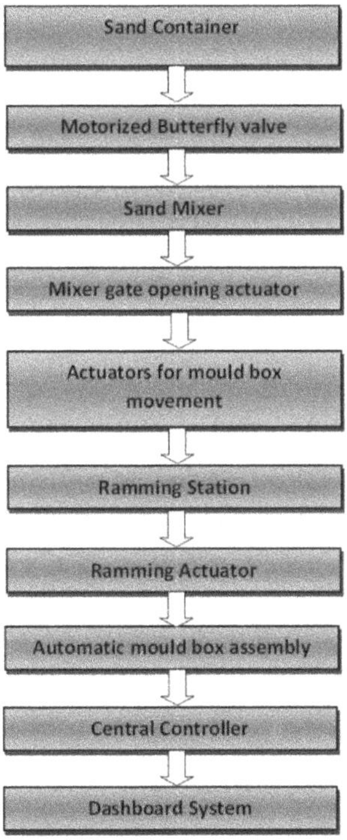

Figure AIV.16 Operational steps for SMART FOUNDRY.

filled up manually in the container which has a butterfly-type valve for regulating the sand quantity to be poured into the mixer. A pump is used to discharge the hardener into the mixer. The pneumatic actuators are used for releasing the sand into the mold box. Then, the movement for the ramming station is provided accordingly. Subsequently, the mold box is automatically opened and the mold is brought with the help of the mold box assembly and the mold box gate is automatically closed for proper functionality. This is operated through a central controller. The operation steps are shown in Figure AIV.16.

Data sensing and analytics: Under this part, a visual dashboard is developed for real-time monitoring of the entire operation through a computer or a smart phone. All process parameters and other relevant data are collected from all physical subsystems, streamed to the cloud and displayed on the mentioned dashboard. Data analysis software is also connected with the dashboard for analysis of process data.

By developing this foundry system, IoT-enabled technology having smart features (Industry 4.0 concept) have been created. This provides machine-to-machine communication and can be trained to take self-decision that reduces human intervention. With this example, it can be said that the concept of Industry 4.0 in smart manufacturing can enhance the overall operational efficiency in an effective manner.

Index

M

O

P

R

S

T

W

Z

For Product Safety Concerns and Information please contact our EU representative GPSR@taylorandfrancis.com
Taylor & Francis Verlag GmbH, Kaufingerstraße 24, 80331 München, Germany

www.ingramcontent.com/pod-product-compliance
Lightning Source LLC
Chambersburg PA
CBHW070716220326
41598CB00024BA/3173